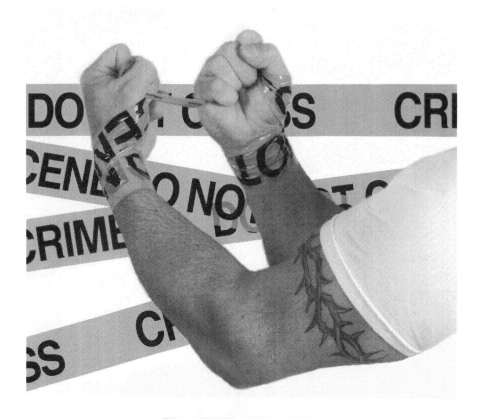

The **RENEGADE'S**
GUIDE
to **Massage Therapy**

A Challenge for Excellence

Robert B. Haase, LMP

Author Photo by Valerie Terrell, Defining Image Photography

Wedding photos by Renee White Photography

Cover photo by Holly Haase

I Want To Thank:

I want to thank my friends and family for their support during this project. My parents, Robert L. and Violet Haase, have been a huge blessing by supporting and encouraging me as well as helping to proofread the early manuscript.

A big thank you to those who helped edit and review the manuscript, including Jessica Hull, Heather Lord, Kris Rose and Monet Smith.

Thanks to Cheryl Fried for her page-by-page insights and feedback, helping to shape the final version.

I want to give special thanks to Tamara Snell who took the time to go through every word of the book with me, several times, helping to create a clear, succinct message that tells my story.

Lastly, I want to thank my three amazing daughters, Ashley, Sara and Holly, who are the light of my eyes and the joy that fills my heart. Their love and support are a huge blessing to me and I am so proud of them as they each embrace their futures with confidence and excitement.

Table of Contents

Forward

Please forgive the stereotype, but you know the type: pocket protector, white tape holding the glasses together, personality only an inanimate computer could love, and inordinate obsession of all things sterile and data-filled. Apt description of a research geek, isn't it? Add in a medical degree and you have all kinds of ego, an alphabet-sized list of initials after the name, and firmly held beliefs based upon layer after layer of theory and tradition. At least this had been my experience working as a nurse at a number of top-notch, research hospitals all across the US.

Do not get me wrong, research is crucial and valuable for providing excellence in healthcare. It has been my privilege to work with some of the top doctors and researchers in my specialty area of intensive care. Often our work set the standards of care for the rest of the country, if not the world.

Achieving a place on those teams and remaining a strong and effective patient & family advocate was a challenge to say the least. More often than not, input from a bedside nurse - especially if it challenged the institution's thinking or traditional way of doing things - was almost regarded as a "clear and present danger." Warnings of CRIME SCENE - DO NOT CROSS were subtly implied. At least until I had opportunity to present my case - with proven skills and knowledge - to the "judge & jury" during grand rounds.

And then I attended a seminar and met Robert Haase,

LMP, a.k.a. Renegade [research] Massage Therapist. He was stylin' with a Charlie Sheen bowling shirt, disarming smile and entertaining personality. So much for fitting into a stereotype! He was also an articulate, funny, and riveting speaker who actually *encouraged* people to challenge what he was saying. His passion for teaching and challenging therapists to be excellent was refreshing and inspiring!

However there were a number of rather unorthodox ideas and moments which got my stiff-necked, traditional medical training all in an uproar. So I readily accepted his offer to a challenge which quickly became a sparring of ideas - much like the duel between Inigo Montoya (me) and the masked Westley disguised as the Dread Pirate Roberts (our own Renegade Robert) in the movie *The Princess Bride*. My life changed drastically for the better that weekend as we quickly became friends. "Iron sharpens iron, so a friend sharpens a friend" (Proverbs 27:16 NLT) has proven to be true for us, just as it did for Inigo & Westley. It has been my distinct privilege to work alongside Robert as a seminar assistant, collaborate on continuing education projects and client case studies, and now with the editing of this, his first book. Because I was willing to accept his challenge to pursue excellence, I have become a much better massage therapist, nurse, business owner and friend.

Will you accept his challenge for excellence? Your life and business will never be the same. En garde, my friend!

- Tamara Jeayne Snell, BSN, RN, AAS, CMT

My Vision: The Future of Massage

Mary had just won her age bracket in the Hawaiian Ironman competition. She was full of laughter and vigor. Her silver hair was short and spiked and her voice could be heard reverberating through the halls of the health club. Mary was larger than life.

When she arrived for her first massage at my clinic, Mary simply said, "Work me over - deep. I just finished the Ironman and I need a good massage. Make sure you really work my legs."

When I pulled back the sheet to reveal the 67-year old woman's muscular leg, it was literally covered with varicose veins. I flashed back to my massage school training and said, "I can't massage your legs."

Mary lifted her head off of the table and looked me in the eye with one eyebrow raised. "Why the hell not?!" Her voice hovered at a growl.

I squinted as I spoke with reduced assurance... "Uh, you have a lot of varicose veins."

With an evenly paced voice and slight agitation, she responded, "What's your point?"

"I could throw a clot if I work on your legs and cause stroke, paralysis or death." My voice became less assured.

"Think I got a clot, do ya??" she said with a slightly sarcastic tone. "Look, I just got back from Hawaii where I swam 2.4 miles, raced my bike 112 miles and then followed it up with a full marathon in less than 8-hours. If I had a clot, I'd be dead. Now massage my damn legs!"

It was at that moment that I realized what I had been

taught in school might not be entirely true. Sometimes you have to ask, "why?" Why are we being told the information that the teacher states as truth? Do they teach out of fear or confidence? Who says what they teach is actual fact? Or is it just an opinion? Is it based on anatomy, conjecture, or worse yet, old information being retold as perpetuated myth?

My focus in life changed that day. I started asking "why?" much more than I had in the past. Mary is one of the inspirations that not only led to my challenging the status quo and beginning my own research for the advancement of the massage profession, but also the writing of this book.

I suppose this book really should begin with my vision, or dream, for our profession. Trying to teach or manage massage therapists was once described to me as "like trying to herd cats." It just cannot be done. Why? We are all very different. Massage therapists have different beliefs, different training and different touch. People become massage therapists for a plethora of reasons. With so many therapists having such divergent belief systems and motivations, how is it possible for me to have a united vision for such a dis-united profession? That is simple…

> ### *My dream is for excellence.*

It is my hope that every massage therapist is excellent at what they do. When you break a bone and go to a hospital, you do not wonder, "Geez… I hope the doctors know how to reset my bone." You *assume* they know how. Yet when we schedule a massage with an unknown therapist, while on vacation, most of us think, "I hope this massage doesn't suck." It is not the best idea for all therapists' styles to be the same, but they should all be exceptional if the public is ever going to trust our profession.

I have been accused of "not believing" in energy work. *YES*, I believe in energy work. Does electricity heal us? Yes. An AED (Automatic External Defibrillator) can bring someone out of ventricular fibrillation. Can electricity kill us? Yes. Ask a lineman working for the electric company. That said, if you paid to learn an energy-based technique that taught you how to "read" and "alter" someone's energy over the course of a weekend, you got taken. You are not feeling what you think you are feeling.

I once asked an internationally-renowned educator of craniosacral therapy seminars a question.

"If I asked ten students, who trained in one of your craniosacral therapy seminars, to evaluate what they 'felt' when touching the same client, how many would feel the same thing and give the same assessment?"

Sheepishly, he replied, "None."

If the nuances of touch involving a physiological condition are difficult to perceive, how much more would the "energetic" be difficult to perceive? Is it possible? Absolutely. That said, it takes most therapists years to hone their palpation skills to that level.

Rick Niemeyer, a teacher at the massage school I founded (the Bodymechanics School of Myotherapy & Massage), used to repeat the mantra, "10,000 massages, Grasshopper", to our students on a regular basis. Rick was on to something. It takes time to learn not just *how* to touch, but to *know* what it is that you are actually feeling. My hope is that therapists will stop "visualizing" what they are feeling based on nonsensical "feelings" of reality and get out an anatomy book to truly understand the more probable reality.

> *We all have the <u>ability</u> to be*
> *exceptional, but we need to truly*
> *make that our desire as well.*

One of the dangers in educating massage therapists is giving them the false understanding of what it means to "assess" a client. Too often we become diagnosticians, believing that we are to diagnose a client's condition. That is not within our scope of practice.

I went to a continuing education class that taught massage therapists how to use a goniometer to measure leg-length discrepancies and how to document that information. What are we to do with that knowledge? Can I tell a client that his right leg is 1.5cm shorter than his left leg? No. That would be diagnosing. Nor can I say, "Sir, you need to go get a full shoe shim to accommodate the leg length difference"... again, still diagnosing. All I am able to do, after meticulously measuring the client's angles and distances between bony landmarks, is refer them to a physician for evaluation. All I can simply say is, "I have some concerns that you may have potential issues which could be affecting your body's posture and causing dysfunction. I suggest you see a physician for an evaluation."

My point is, if the doctor is going to diagnose the

condition anyway, your evaluation should be cursory at best, lest you fall into the realm of diagnosing. It is not just a matter of semantics. A massage therapist's assessment is not intended for the diagnosis of pathologies.

> *It is this simple: If something hurts when you touch it, it probably has a problem. Healthy tissue does not hurt when you touch it.*

As therapists, it is our job to refer out as necessary for the client's benefit. I often hear about massage therapists selling their clients herbal concoctions from a network marketing company rather than referring them to a doctor for evaluation of their condition. Sometimes that condition ends up actually being cancer. Other times, therapists suggest exercises for a client's shoulder "weakness" when it is actually a torn labrum. Again, we need to stick to our scope of practice and feel comfortable operating within those parameters.

Massage therapists need to come to terms that we cannot be specialists in all fields. As Yoda might say, "A year in massage school does not a doctor make." Just saying.

Again, do I want every therapist to be the same? By no means. I do, however, want us all to provide exceptional care so that when clients pay their hard-earned money for a massage, they receive something that is extraordinary. My hope is that the client receives amazing touch, backed by solid knowledge, and accurate information based on sound anatomy and physiologically. Not a bunch of "new-age-mumbo-jumbo-cosmic-energy." If it is, the technique had better provide consistent and verifiable results.

As massage therapists, we have the power to affect change in this world, and to affect people's health and quality of life. Bottom line, massage therapy is not a job, but a calling. Stop making money your goal and start changing lives!

Each of us is shaped, in one way or another, by the experiences of our past. Shaped both in good and bad ways. Experiences do not shape reality, but affect how we see and interpret reality. Therapists must understand the difference. A good personal injury attorney will tell you that if he has several witnesses to the same collision, each witness may interpret what they saw differently, arriving at different conclusions.

For example, if every time your mother makes chocolate chip cookies there is a simultaneous earthquake somewhere in the world, you should not blame the cookies. Coincidences observed should take a back seat to experience that imparts wisdom. When I think back to how I came to believe what I do and what has made me a successful massage therapist, I am amazed how the smallest of experiences have made the biggest impact.

> *Renegade Revelation:*
> *Life lessons are only valuable if we*
> *learn from them. And the lesson is*
> *not always what we first perceive,*
> *but often lies deeper.*

This book is divided into three parts. First, the life lessons, or *"Renegade Revelations"* that I have gleaned beginning with my first job as a paperboy, through my years in business, massage therapy and school ownership. Second, are the *Renegade Revelations* that I discovered through bodywork that will give you insights to help you with your own practice. Third, I will discuss some of the "Perpetuated Myths" that continue to persist throughout the massage profession.

The fact that you are reading this book likely means you are looking to improve yourself within your profession. Even if you are not a massage therapist and are in another line of work, you will gain some valuable business insights that can easily be applied to your profession. Truth is truth, regardless of how it is learned.

Life Before Massage Therapy

My Early Years

I remember when I was in the 6th grade and our neighborhood paperboy stopped by my house to ask if I wanted a job. "It's easy", he said. "Plus, you can make good money!"

I was so excited to take on his newspaper customers as my own. In today's dollars, I made over $300.00 a month for flinging the newspaper onto 70+ doorsteps, 7-afternoons a week. That paper route taught me about responsibility, collection with accounts payable, inventory, paying bills, hiring temporary workers, and being on-time (calls came into the house if the paper was late.) That is huge for a 12-year old.

The first summer I was told that I had to attend a mandatory "training week" at *The Daily Olympian* newspaper circulation offices. That is when I met the circulation manager, Ron Hill, a man who soon taught me unique insights into business, finance and success.

I was stunned by the shelves of cool prizes that would be given to kids who made the most subscription sales. Bicycles, gas-powered remote control airplanes, camping gear, knives... I was awestruck. I *wanted* those toys. All I had to do was sell subscriptions. Piece of cake, right?

I ventured into my neighborhood and knocked on lots of doors. But every time I asked people if they wanted to subscribe to the newspaper, they would just say, "NO", and shut the door in my face. My mother saw that I was a little disillusioned from my lack of success and told me to call Steve Shorb, a family friend. He had been a paperboy years before and apparently had exceptional sales skills.

Steve picked me up on a Saturday morning and drove me to an apartment complex in Olympia, Washington. We got out of the car and Steve said, "Let's see what you've got!"

I knocked on the first door. A woman answered my knock.

"Do you take *The Daily Olympian* newspaper, ma'am?"

"No", she replied.

"Would you like to?"

"No", she replied, half-smiled, and then she shut the door.

Steve looked at me with scrunched-up eyebrows and snapped, "What was that?!"

"She said 'no'", I said sheepishly.

Steve said, "You got the right answer to the wrong question. Watch." Then he proceeded to knock on the door again! I was so embarrassed.

The woman opened the door with a "What now?!" look on her face and Steve said, "Ma'am, I'm sorry, my friend here didn't tell you about the paper and why you can't live without it."

"I don't want it", she sighed as she began to shut the door again. The door bounced off of Steve's well-placed foot, which kept the door from closing fully.

"Why is that?" Steve quizzed.

"I can't afford it."

Steve got a big smile on face. "Ma'am! You can't afford *not* to take the paper! You'll save several times the cost with the coupons that you find in the paper each week. You'll actually *make* money with the paper!"

—

18

With each excuse, Steve had a response as to why they actually could not do without the paper. Then he followed, "Would you prefer that the delivery start next Monday or on Wednesday, our big 'coupon day'?"

"Wednesday", she responded. I was stunned. Steve did not just ask if she wanted the daily paper, but had responses that made sense when he heard each of her objections.

I was one of the top three subscription sales-boys for four years, earning what is now the equivalent of over $800.00 per week during the summer months. My father not only told me, at the age of 12, that I was now to buy my own clothes and pay for my activities, but actually asked to borrow some money from me. Thank you, Steve Shorb, for the valuable lesson you taught me.

> *Renegade Revelation:*
> *You need to know <u>why</u> your client or customer <u>needs</u> to have your product. If your product is not so amazing that they absolutely <u>must</u> have it, you are offering the wrong product.*

Shortly after I entered high school, a fellow drummer asked if I was looking for work. "They're hiring at the Sizzler", he said with a smile.

What an awesome opportunity! By the way, this is back in the late 1970's when Sizzler was still a bona fide steakhouse. I was hired as a busboy. Within a year and a half I was making union, chef wages as the backup head cook. As a junior in high school I was making $22.00 an hour in 2012 dollars. Holy crap! I was rolling in money! At the same time, I had this sense of dread that I was doing a job that was leading nowhere - at least nowhere near where I eventually wanted to be.

At the time, I was also the advertising editor for our high school's award-winning newspaper. I wanted to get into marketing and advertising as a career one day so flipping steaks was not exactly on the path to my dream job.

In the days leading up to my final night in charge at the Sizzler, our lead chef and prep cook had been smoking enough weed in the back room to make a steroid-enraged, professional wrestler become mellow. Thanks to the pot, the chef forgot to order steaks for the days ahead.

My shift started at 3:30pm that Thursday night and I was left in charge while both the restaurant manager and lead chef went home. When I looked into the meat coolers it was clear that something was wrong... there were not enough entree items! Crap. Around 5:00pm, I told the waitstaff that we were out of top sirloin steaks and to let the customers know if they ordered one. At 5:15pm, we were out of New York steaks. At 5:30pm, no more chicken cordon bleu and no more filet mignon. We were embarrassing ourselves.

As each person ordered their meal, the staff had to inform them that we did not have what they wanted. That is death to any business.

I made a judgment call at 5:45pm. I told the staff, "Close it down. No more customers will be served regardless of what they order... turn on the "closed" sign."

The next day I got "ripped a new one" by the manager, but I stood by my decision as I explained that I had no choice. I handed him my key as I said, "I'm not destined to be a cook anyway, and I certainly don't want your job when I grow up. It's been nice to have known you."

I walked out the door with my integrity intact deciding I would rather work in retail sales, even though most jobs for teenagers at shopping malls paid less than half of what I made as a chef. The upside would be that I would not smell like grease when I got home and I would be on a path towards attaining my goals. Learning to sell retail? Right direction. Flipping steaks? Wrong direction.

> *Renegade Revelation:*
> *Making a high wage is an obstacle*
> *to happiness if you are not doing*
> *what you are meant to be doing.*

The very next day, after leaving The Sizzler, I went to the local shopping mall to apply for a job at Mr. Rags. It was *the* place to buy clothes if you were a teenage boy. I was immediately hired (must have been my hair).

Only a week after starting, the manager mysteriously left the company and the new manager told me that he was going to have let me go. Not because I was not doing a great job of selling, but because a girl named Lucy had to be rehired. It seems the recently-departed manager fired her because she would not put up with his unwanted sexual advances. I said, "Of course you

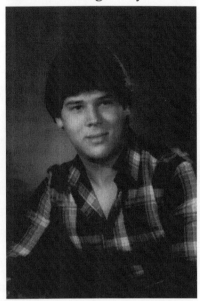

Me, with hair. Circa 1980.

should rehire her. I completely understand." So the next day I went to the Mr. Rags store in a neighboring city and hoped to convince the manager that I should be hired. Although he would not know who I was, I figured I was qualified.

As I entered the store on a quiet weekday morning, the manager at the front register was on the phone in what seemed like an important conversation. So important that he did not say a word to me, just nodded to acknowledge my presence. I stood patiently on the other side of the store and waited. It was obvious that he was working by himself. As I waited, a man walked up to me from the other side of the store and asked, "Do these pants go well with this shirt?" I smiled and said, "Yes! And let me show you how you can make this work even better..."

I proceeded to lead the customer around the store from rack to rack and showed him how to take just a few items and create many great outfits. When he seemed pleased with his new wardrobe, we approached the cash register as the manager ended his call. "Can you 'ring this guy up' for me?" I asked with a half-smile, half-grin. After the manager finished the sale and sent the customer on his way he said, "So, when can you start?"

> *Renegade Revelation:*
> *Learn to recognize opportunity*
> *and do not hesitate to act with*
> *boldness.*

After working for Mr. Rags, I received an opportunity to become the youngest person to ever sell men's suits at the local Bon Marche (now Macy's). It was an increase in pay and a better work environment. I was set. After my initial training, I was put onto the sales floor. While I was trained in Seattle, my job was in Olympia. What a difference 60-miles makes. I did not realize that 60-miles could take you back in time 10-years although I am told the difference between Chicago, Illinois and Des Moines, Iowa is about 30-years. That is up for debate in Midwest pubs, but I am getting off-topic. It seemed the Olympia store was the place that the company buyers sent all of the clothing that the other stores could not sell. While "dickeys" (a fake turtle neck that was tucked under the collar of a dress shirt) were popular in the 1960's and early 70's, they were not worn in the early 80's. The Seattle buyers at the Bon did not know that though. Much of the clothing sold at a crawl from our department until I convinced the department manager to let me contact the buyers directly. A few short discussions later and we were moving product. It was not that difficult.

> *Renegade Revelation:*
> *Do not sell what you have. Sell what the customer needs. If they do not know they need it, educate them. If they do not need it, get a product that they do need.*

After working in retail sales at several clothing stores, I came to understand what it meant to work for a living versus making an income. I remember opening a box of shirts from a manufacturer while working at the a department store. The box included a packing slip that showed the retail price and the wholesale cost. The shirts sold for $60.00, but the wholesale cost was only $15.00! Seriously? I took 5-minutes to sell the shirt, was paid less than a dollar for my labor and the store cleared over $44.00. Granted, they had overhead and advertising to pay, but wow! While working at another store, I remember selling a customer a whole new wardrobe. I made just $3.00 for my time, but the store cleared over $700.00 in profit, before overhead. It was at that point I realized that I was going about this "income" thing entirely wrong.

Within a few weeks, I found a way to buy home and car audio equipment wholesale, rather than make a couple of dollars selling for someone else. I could sell one sound system a week out of my home and make as much money, if not more, than if I worked a full week for someone else. I quit my job and sold audio equipment throughout my college years.

> *Renegade Revelation:*
> *Work Less. Make more. (Work*
> *smart, not hard.)*

I named my new company Silverwind Enterprises. At first, I was excited just to get a sale. But word spread quickly about my fair prices, which included personal installation and setup. Business grew rapidly. I could buy a car stereo for $80.00 wholesale and then sell it for $199.00, which was below the competition. The problem was I charged a profit that felt "right" at the moment. I did not write those prices down. So the first time two people, who had purchased the same car stereo from me, spoke to each other, I had a problem. One of them called up and said, "You overcharged me! Why did Kerry get the same thing for $50.00 less?!"

> *Renegade Revelation:*
> *Have a pricing strategy and stick to it.*

My Adult Years

While in college, I received a phone call from Mike Daniels who worked with one of the wholesale companies from which I bought electronics. He said that he would like to meet for lunch. When we met, Mike spent a few minutes complimenting me on my small business and asked if I would be interested in coming to work for the distributor over my Christmas and summer breaks. I tried to convince him that I was not looking for a job, but he ended up winning at the "convincing game." Not only was the job going to pay me well, plus commissions, it kept me on my career track in sales and marketing. I remembered my earlier revelation to make decisions that bring me closer to my goal, so I agreed and ended up working for the company over summer and winter breaks throughout college. While making good money with the company, it was clear that the corporate world was *not* in my DNA.

After college, I briefly worked as a district manager for the same newspaper for whom I had delivered papers as a boy. Later I moved on to a job in Lynnwood, Washington, as a marketing assistant for a company that built "pole building" garages, barns and riding arenas.

In just three months I was promoted from marketing assistant to sales manager. At first I was overwhelmed since I was only a 23-year old kid managing a sales team of 35 to 55-year old men. The skills that I had learned in my early years helped increase sales from 45 buildings a month to around 90 a month. With one inquiry from our "Little Nickel" advertisements, our salesmen could make one appointment, with one potential customer, and sell the building 50% of the time. How? The salesman answered the customer's questions and met their needs while overcoming obstacles and dissolving objections.

How do you get 90 buildings sold in one month? First, you use an advertisement that compels the potential customer to call. Second, when they call, you do not just give information over the phone, but make an appointment to meet face-to-face. Thus increasing the number of potential buyers to whom you can sell. Third, you increase the "closing rate" of sales from 30% to 50%, using solid communication techniques.

> *Renegade Revelation:*
> *Make your advertizing compelling and give the customer a reason to call.*

> *Renegade Revelation:*
> *Find a way to meet with the customer face-to-face because people hire* _people_*, rather than voices or advertisements.*

> *Renegade Revelation:*
> *Clearly communicate what you can and cannot do and solve any problem or obstacle that arises.*

After two intense years, I left the pole-building/ residential metal building field. I would explain the reason I use the description "intense", but it is the premise of an entire book I could write about business owners and how they manage the management... perhaps someday.

I was hired by a commercial steel building company that built structures for companies like Boeing and Kenworth Trucks. These were big, expensive structures. When I was hired, the owner said, "Here is a list of all the buildings we have built over the past 30-years. I would like you to take this map book and go look at all of them over the next month."

I asked, "Don't you want me to sell something?"

"Nope", he quipped. "We just want you to get to know our product first."

"How soon are you expecting me to make my first sale?"

He put his hand to his chin, as to think deeply, and said, "Well, if you don't make a sale after a year, we can talk about it and see what might be going wrong."

A year?! They were going to pay me to drive around, talk to folks and *maybe* sell something? The manager continued, "This is the commercial steel building business. No quick sales here. You're in it for the long-sale. You take your time, build relationships, build trust, and help the customer to see why they are investing their company's money to buy a very expensive product from us. We are the most expensive company out there, but what we provide is second to none."

The point was that it was not about low prices or how fast you could get someone to relinquish their money.

> *Renegade Revelation:*
> *Build relationships, provide*
> *quality, and charge handsomely*
> *for it. Quick and cheap is for other*
> *businesses with lesser standards.*

After several years in the commercial steel building business, I felt unrest in my heart about what I was doing with my life. I made good money, worked for a great company, had a nice home and a nice car with an awesome wife and baby. What more could I want? I had the American dream… right? Not so much. At the end of my day, my wife would ask me, "What did you do today?" My answer was nearly always the same: "Well, I put together some preliminary structural drawings, prepared a couple of estimates, took a potential customer to lunch and signed a few contracts." Her response? "Oh, okay."

I thought about the ironworkers that spent their days constructing buildings. When they got home, what did their wife or significant other get as a response to that same question? The worker would likely say, "I BUILT THAT!" It was official. I was jealous of guys in hard hats. Not because of their job, but because their productivity led to long-lasting results. God forbid, but if our economy was to dissolve during a complete. international meltdown, which would bring our country to financial ruin, what could I offer if bartering was the only method of value exchange? What skills did I really have to offer this world? I could sell something, right? Ugh. I wanted so much more. I wanted to make a difference in people's lives with something meaningful that did not require anything other than my own two hands.

Meanwhile, playing in the back of my mind was the realization that I had already achieved my career goals just a few years out of college. Sounds impressive, does it? Not so much. Here were my goals:

1. Make more money than my father
2. Live in the Redmond/Bellevue area and own a home there (considered the seat of success at the time because of Microsoft, Nintendo, etc)
3. Own a Volvo 740 Inter-cooled Turbo, advertised as being as fast as a Porsche 944

Yes, those were shallow goals, but to a college student, they were huge. When I attained them so quickly, I realized that my goals were shallow and meaningless. I wanted something more that had deeper, lasting value.

Late one night, I found myself watching an old, black and white movie when I could not sleep. Two men were conversing while on adjacent tables receiving massage in a men's club. I kept looking at the men massaging them. They looked like Mr. Clean wearing khaki slacks, white tee-shirt and shaved heads. *I* could do that. I took out my phonebook and looked for massage schools (it was 1989... we still used phonebooks).

Within a few days, I discovered the Brian Utting School of Massage, called them, enrolled in an all-day, introductory workshop and made an appointment for a tour.

The school was located not far from the Space Needle in downtown Seattle. It was old, made of brick, had creaky wooden stairs and lots of live plants. When I met with

Marlene, the woman who gave me the official tour, I knew this school really was not for me. It was probably great for hippies, but I was a man with a pressed-white shirt, Nordstrom tie and shiny Volvo. It even had one of the first built-in cell phones with the cool curly-cord that stretched from the phone to the dash. I was *not* a hippie. Besides, Brian's brochure consisted of just a few pages, simply formatted on a Mackintosh computer, printed with black ink on plain white paper and stapled at the corner. I was not impressed. But I wanted to see if massage was for me, so I decided to register for the school's one-day, introductory workshop.

When the day of the workshop arrived, I was a little unsettled. There were a *lot* of naked people. I still have this image of the teacher as he dropped his clothing to the floor and gracefully got onto the massage table in front of everyone! Then, women took off their clothes and climbed casually onto the tables when it was their turn. Nobody seemed to be in a rush. There were naked body parts everywhere. That was new for me. I had to seriously concentrate on what I was doing that day. I started to question myself. "Can I do this? Can I go to massage school when people are walking around naked? How am I supposed to learn anything with all of this nakedness??!!" I needed to take the class again to make sure I could separate the nudity from my learning process. Thankfully I could (Official Note: Brian changed the "nudity policy" shortly thereafter.).

Despite my discomfort, it became clear that I was being called to become a massage therapist. The idea of helping people, using my hands and relieving pain was appealing. This was *it*! When I told my wife that I wanted to give up my

"Bellevue/Redmond" life and go back to school to become a poor, massage therapist, she simply said, "Uh... okay." Then it was time to tell my family.

I asked my parents to join us for dinner one Sunday. After we finished eating, we all sat in the living room. I took a deep breath and told my parents that I could not continue in a job that was not fulfilling and I felt that massage therapy was what I was supposed to be doing with my life. I will never forget what my father said to me next.

Dad's face got serious. "Bob, I've been an accountant for the past 30-years and I've hated every minute of it... do what makes you happy."

And that was that. I was going back to school. I took a leap of faith and quit my unsatisfying job.

> *Renegade Revelation:*
> *Risk doing what you are called to*
> *do. Trust your calling.*

It was time to find a good massage school, so I started by requesting information from the biggest school in Washington State. It was well known and well funded. The brochure was slick and glossy with photos that were taken professionally. As an advertising and marketing guy, I was impressed.

I then visited a smaller school. It was located in a series of old homes in Tacoma, Washington. It was a good school, but more "spa" based than what I wanted and it did not feel like a good fit for me, so I kept looking.

Uncertain of where to get my education, I ended up going back for another meeting with Marlene at the Brian Utting School. It still did not feel as professional as I thought it should be – after all, his brochure was plain black and white versus full-color and glossy. The big school was where I had to go.

I had just completed the school's application and had fee in hand when I received a call from Marlene at Brian's school. She wanted to know if she could expect my application. I told her that I had chosen the big school. She said, "Bob, please, before you do that, can you meet with Brian personally? One-on-one. He wants you here and I know you'll be glad you talked with him."

I figured I had nothing to lose. I would let him down easily without being disrespectful about his unprofessional information packet or make him feel bad that his school did not stack up to the competition's professionalism. At least that was my plan.

When I walked in the door to meet with Brian, he had this calm peace about him. As he greeted me, he shook my hand and had me sit in an adjacent chair. He had a thin, frail frame, chiseled features and his hair slicked back into a ponytail. I could see why the school felt like a hippie haven. Brian looked like a hippie who was trying to look professional. Looks can be deceiving.

It is amazing how the outward appearance can be easily peeled back when immense wisdom, caring and focus emerges from deep within. Brian opened his mouth and began to speak. He asked me about my goals, my dreams, and my desires for the future. He then proceeded to tell me about his philosophy of bodywork, how he started teaching, why his school creates excellent graduates and why he did not just feel - but *knew* - he could teach me to be the best, more so than any other school. Those stapled sheets of paper became irrelevant. Brian was a living, breathing representation of the heart of the Brian Utting School.

I tossed the Seattle school's application and enrolled in Brian's school full-time in the fall of 1990. I am grateful that I woke up from that other, hypnotizing brochure which initially grabbed my attention. Brian would later deliver on his promise. Amidst an insanely-diverse group of students and a plethora of eccentric teachers, I would eventually emerge with the skills to succeed. Thank you, Brian.

> *Renegade Revelation:*
> *Presentation is not everything. A*
> *sexy car without an engine is*
> *worthless compared to a dull and*
> *unpainted Ferrari. Be excellent vs.*
> *flashy.*

With no desire to continue in the steel building field, I quit my job six months before school was to start. I decided to fill the void by working for a Jenny Craig diet center where I taught nutrition classes and worked with clients that were not so adept at following the diet plan. I was the "hard-ass" diet counselor. If you were morbidly obese and not sticking to the plan, you got Bob Haase, "The Fixer." It was my job to "scare 'em straight."

While working at Jenny Craig, I was able to conduct my first health experiment. I blame my experimentation tendencies on my mother. Let me explain.

Back in my junior high school years, my mother was attempting to concoct *the* ultimate cheesecake recipe. Every other night or so, mom had a new cheesecake for the family to try after dinner. She experimented for about a month until she finally figured it out. She found *the* one recipe that everyone agreed was the best. As I watched each cheesecake bake in the oven, I had no idea that the temperature dial on the oven would be the key to my success as a therapist one day.

Fast forward to the diet center where I had my "cheesecake" moment. I decided to have half of my clients agree to drink a full gallon of water and the other half to drink only a half-gallon, daily. Surprisingly, those that drank a gallon a day lost weight at twice the speed of those who did not. My experimentation began. Thanks, Mom.

It was time to leave Jenny Craig and become a full-time student again.

> *Renegade Revelation:*
> *Compare and experiment to find*
> *what works best.*

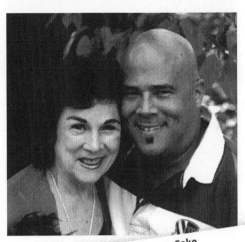

Mom's Favorite Cheese Cake

Crust—make and set aside:
(Use Spring form pan)
   1 Cup Graham Cracker crumbs
   3 Tbsp. Sugar
   ¼ tsp. cinnamon
   3 Tbsp. Melted butter

Fillings:
      Cream together:
         2 tsp. lemon peal
         3 8 oz. cream cheese (24 oz,)

      Add:
         1 cup sugar
         ¼ tsp. salt.
         5 Large eggs (Use eggs that
         are room temperature)

Blend all three on Medium speed
      Then beat 10 minutes.

      Pour filling into crust, bake at 350-
degrees for 45-minutes.
      Cool 20 minutes

Top Layer:
      Beat:
         1 ½ cups sour cream
         ½   tsp. vanilla
         2 Tbsp. sugar

         Mix and spread all three over cake
         Bake at 350-degrees for 10-
         minutes
         Cool & chill

My Massage School Year

My year at the Brian Utting School had a huge impact on my life in numerous ways. I could actually write a book specifically about that experience alone, but for now will focus on this book and what has led me to become a Renegade Massage Therapist.

The underlying theme of my entire massage school experience came down to a one-word mantra: *Why*? It seems I asked that word a lot, almost excessively. I can think of no other profession or segment of society that has a "they said it, so it must be true" mentality more than massage therapy. And, that includes multi-level/network marketing companies (e.g.: *"This exclusive product with our proprietary formula cures cancer in just 2-weeks!"*)

While in school, we were constantly told "truths" about massage and it's benefits. The problem was it was misinformation being retold from teacher to student. When that student became a teacher, the cycle continued. All massage schools were guilty of the same thing to some degree - some more than others.

One day, a chiropractor/bodyworker and founder of a large naturopathic college came to speak to our class. He was treated as a demigod - at least in the eyes of most of my fellow students. During his lecture, someone asked how to feel "energy" while performing bodywork. He told the students, "I want you to hold your arms out in front of you. Now, pull your hands back into extension as hard as you can. Pull hard! Hold it... extend as hard as you can... hold it for 2-minutes..." After the two-minutes had passed, he said, "Now, I want you to relax your arms and then bring your palms together, but do not let them touch. Bounce them gently... bringing them towards each other and away from each other. Do you feel that resistance as you do that? Feel the gentle repulsion of the palms resisting each other? *That* is energy! You're feeling energy!"

I raised my hand, and patiently waited for the chiropractor to call on me. "Yes?" he said.

"BULLSHIT!", I emphatically exclaimed. "We aren't feeling energy at all. What we are feeling is the tension that has built up from causing our forearm muscles to go into spasm and fatigue. That over-stretched position caused enough fatigue to make it appear that there was a force between our palms, but it isn't energy, just fatigue."

He stammered, "Well, okay... it isn't energy. But, it *feels* like energy!"

"Then don't tell us an untruth to make us believe something that isn't so." As those words left my lips, my class was sure of it - I had angered the gods and it might not be wise to sit near me any longer.

As my school education progressed, my mantra morphed from "why?" to "how do you know that to be true?" and "is this true and replicable in most cases?" As massage therapists, we are still in the relative infancy of our profession. The medical profession is looking for continuity, congruency, efficacy and most of all, sanity in our thoughts. When massage therapists put "belief" above fact and perpetuate myths that border on the absurd, we come across as uneducated.

Consistently, there was a theme of faulty logic being demonstrated in my fellow students as they discussed what they felt were "realities" and "truth." For example, they felt that acupuncture healed their sinuses and the fact that they were on a course of antibiotics was purely coincidental. Or, they were convinced by a network marketer that a certain brand of magnets can cure scoliosis overnight. I think my favorite was a fellow student that tried to convince the rest of the class that smoking marijuana puts a special coating on the surface of your lung tissue that filters and protects you from environmental toxins and disease.

It didn't help that some of our "profession's best" came and taught nonsensical things, like, "My massage clinic has spirits that take care of me. They even fill my oil bottle at night." My fellow students squirmed when I asked, "Do you happen to have a cleaning person that works at your clinic after hours?"

"Yes, why do you ask?" she asked with a puzzled face.

"No reason." I grinned.

The philosophy of "if they say it, it must be true" was even more present when the students would be preparing to practice a new technique on the chest or abdomen and our instructor would say, "Don't be surprised if you experience an emotional release during your practice time today. It is completely normal and very common. Many of you will experience emotional release today." I will discuss the power of suggestion later in this book, but for now, suffice it to say that if the teacher put that thought into the student's fertile minds, it *would* happen. Later, if we worked on the abdomen and the teacher forgot to mention a potential emotional release, it would seldom happen. Although emotional release is indeed a potential outcome of deep bodywork, keep in mind the power of suggestion is a powerful tool.

One of the habits that helped me most in school was to

go beyond the minimum-required practice hours that the program required. In general, I put in 15-hours each week practicing massage on fellow students, professional massage therapists and "professional receivers" of massage as well. I could not charge for massage, so those that received free work from me had to allow me to not just improve my skills with the school's techniques, but the techniques I was making up on my own as well.

Sadly, receiving massage from many of the licensed massage professionals in my area gave me more lessons about what *not* to do rather than what to do. I actually had a therapist eat a sandwich while she massaged me and allowed her cats to run free and brush along my body during a massage.

At the Brian Utting School, we were given the option to augment our training with a 6-week course in cadaver anatomy at the Bastyr School of Naturopathic Medicine. Wanting to learn all I could, I opted-in.

Over the duration of the course, it was great to have a chance to see inside the body, however, the experience left me more frustrated than anything. If you have never had the opportunity to participate in a cadaver course, then you cannot fully comprehend what I experienced. Please forgive the comparison, but if I handed you a piece of top sirloin steak in one hand and a piece of beef jerky in the other and then told you that the two were the same, you would give me that "what are you talking about?" look. Beef jerky meets "Alien Autopsy" from the 1980's. Google it. Bottom line, it was like looking at a road map versus an actual road. I wanted more.

In the end, my massage school experience taught me

not only how to be an excellent massage therapist, but what I ought not to do as well. Ultimately, it prepared me to eventually create an even better educational experience for my future students and launched me on the path to the most amazing career I could have ever imagined. Thank you, Brian… for everything.

Random Revelations from my Years in Practice

When you see a dentist, they tell you to come back in 6-months for a follow-up/cleaning. When you see a medical doctor or chiropractor, they tell you when to return for optimal benefit. But massage therapists? Most are afraid to tell their clients when they should return or which treatment frequency to suggest for their clients. Who knows the most about the cumulative benefits of massage and the most beneficial frequency of *your* techniques? That would be you. If you do not lead your client with confident suggestions, the competition will.

> *Renegade Revelation:*
> *Clients want to be led through the*
> *healing process.*

If you are massaging a client but do not explain *why* you are doing *what* you are doing, you can confuse the client. For example, when a client presents with suboccipital headaches and you begin treating his pectoralis minor muscles, he will think you are not listening to his complaint. If you explain the correlation between the headache and the antagonistic struggle, which leads to the eventual headache, he will get onboard with your suggested treatment plan and more likely become a "compliant client." Teach and educate your clients. It makes you the expert. People pay more for experts.

> *Renegade Revelation:*
> *Clients want to be educated.*

In the same vein as educating, communication is paramount to your success. If I do not explain why I am working on an area of the body that is completely different than what was asked for, clients will not return. They will tell their friends, "He didn't listen to what I wanted." Be clear, educate and get permission before working on areas that the client did not ask for or expect. Make sure that you also get permission while the client is alert and understanding of what you are asking. Trust me. Asking someone while they are in a drowsy, relaxed state, is not the best time to get permission. They would not remember what you asked, let alone understand why you were asking. Massage can put you into a deep state of relaxation. Be careful.

> *Renegade Revelation:*
> *Listen to your client and*
> *communicate with your intent.*
> *Effective communication is*
> *imperative.*

Some clients lie. They lie on their intake forms. They lie when questioned about their medical history. I have had clients withhold the truth about automotive collisions because they did not want the information to be revealed to an insurance company. I have also had clients commit "lies of omission" while others innocently forget significant pieces of their medical history.

For example, while giving a demonstration of a neck treatment sequence in front of a class, it was clear to me that she likely had residual whiplash from some type of neck incident.

"Have you ever been in a car accident?", I asked.

"No."

My hands felt otherwise. "Are you sure? This feels like whiplash."

"I'm sure. No accidents."

There was incongruity between what my hands felt and her denial of injury, but I kept on teaching and demonstrating.

Suddenly, the woman burst into tears. "Oh my god! I was in an accident two years ago! I flew through the windshield of a car and I forgot!"

Trust your hands. Do not call your client a liar. Whether it is a lapse in memory or an outright desire to conceal information, trust what your hands feel and use appropriate caution around what may be an undisclosed pathology.

Communication is imperative. If their intake form does not match up with what you are feeling while you massage them, ask more questions.

Also be aware that clients may not tell their significant others about the gender of the person who provides their massage. If you want to leave voicemails reminding them of their upcoming appointment, make sure you have permission to do so. I was nearly the cause of several divorces and break-ups because of jealous partners and spouses who heard the messages. I have not made reminder calls since my first week as a massage therapist. Lesson learned. With the advent of online scheduling and automated electronic reminders, this can easily become a non-issue in your practice.

—

> *Renegade Revelation:*
> *Clients conceal. Clients forget.*
> *Clients lie.*

The client is not the one calling the shots when they receive treatment from a therapist. Sure, the client can make requests, but just as they are not handed a scalpel to perform their own surgery, they are usually not knowledgeable enough to safely direct treatment. We are trained in our society that "the customer is always right." Not true in healthcare.

As a massage therapist, you know what is best for your client and it is your responsibility to protect clients from themselves. Shortly after I received my license, I filled in for another therapist. One of her regular clients came to see me and he assumed that I could not possibly know much, let alone be as good as the regular therapist. He had me convinced as well. After all, I was new and inexperienced. What could I know? He had been receiving massage for years and "knew" what he needed. When he arrived for his appointment with me, he said, "I want you to work for 30-minutes as deep as you can, and only on this spot..." He was pointing to the mid-belly of his right rhomboid muscle.

"Okay... it's your massage", I said sheepishly.

"Oh, and *no* ice when you're done. I hate ice", he insisted.

For the next half-hour, I proceeded to give him deep work as he requested. "Is this pressure too much?", I would ask. He would always respond the same, "Perfect. It's a 'good hurt.'" He left after I finished his treatment. I was really wishing he had let me work the antagonists, and more importantly, let me ice him afterwards. I knew better. That is my point. I *knew* better.

The next day, Mister "It's a good hurt-no ice" stopped by the clinic utterly pissed. "I'm calling my attorney! I'm going to sue you for malpractice! You gave me nerve damage!" he snapped in a forceful tone. I simply responded, "I should have done what you *needed* versus what you *insisted* upon. And, you needed ice. You'll feel better in 7-days." He did feel better in 7-days and later apologized for his anger. I also apologized for not educating him as I should have.

As promised, he improved and we mended fences. I also learned a vital lesson. I went to school to be good at what I do and that meant something. If the client has more education regarding soft tissue treatment than I do, then I might handle things differently. Maybe. The point is, if I do not know what I am doing more than my clients do, then I am in the wrong profession.

> *Renegade Revelation:*
> *The client is not "the boss" when it*
> *comes to medical treatment.*

During my first years as a therapist, I utilized my mother's "cheesecake" experiment philosophy. I would often try new technique variations, charting efficacious outcomes and recovery rates. I would take one low back technique, for example, and use it on half of my clients and another technique with the other half. I was constantly searching for the "ultimate" technique for each condition with which my clients presented.

In 1992, my second year as a massage therapist, I was feeling really good about my improving skills due to this technique-development process. Until one day, in walked "Dwight" and everything changed.

Dwight arrived at the clinic in a 1950's show car... spotless and lowered to the ground. He also sported a 1950's slicked-back haircut and spoke with a smug New Jersey accent. During his intake interview, he informed me that he had been in a motor vehicle accident. We began his treatment that afternoon.

On his second visit, Dwight's lovely wife and two, sweet daughters dropped him off for his treatment. Dwight gave each a kiss and told his wife he loved her as the three went for a walk. For some reason, Dwight chose that day to tell me that he was having an affair. With great pride he exclaimed, "She's hot!" I set the thought aside, focused, and proceeded with his treatment.

During his next visit, Dwight told me of yet another woman with whom he was having sex. The following visit, he was exuberant about his ability to setup rendezvous with another *two* new women set for the same day. I was becoming a little frustrated with Dwight at this point. I am not one to judge people, but being a serial philanderer is pushing it.

Yet *again*, during a subsequent visit, Dwight told me of another woman. This time, he tried to tell me about his appreciation of her "stellar" figure. As my elbow was gliding up Dwight's erector spinae group, he said, "Her body was amazing! You should see her..."

At that precise moment I decided, I did *not* want to hear about any woman's body with which Dwight was having sex. I increased my elbow pressure to a level which was likely a 9-plus on the pain scale... Dwight could not talk. I grinned. Every time Dwight tried to restart his description of this woman's body, I dug in deeper, causing him to literally become speechless.

Dwight never did get the opportunity to describe the woman's body that day.

The next day, I received a phone call from Dwight. I was a little apprehensive about what he had to say.

"Bob? Hey, it's Dwight. Look, you're not going to believe this, but after your treatment yesterday, I'm PAIN FREE!"

I paused in thought, "Truly, if there is any person that does *not* deserve to be pain-free right now, it is Dwight."

There was a paradigm shift in my thought process that day. Until that point, I had been comparing techniques... essentially ingredients in a recipe. What I had not considered was the "oven temperature" and how long to leave the "ingredients" in the "oven." I had not been comparing frequency, intensity or duration. There was a whole new dimension to my client experimentation now. I had good techniques, but now I needed to determine the optimal recipes for clients to experience a faster recovery. Thank you, Dwight.

Renegade Revelation:
Ingredients need a recipe.

I have watched several therapists go bankrupt from a common misconception. The reality is, going into debt and spending tens of thousands of dollars to create the "ultimate" office/clinic is a huge mistake. People want a warm, clean and comfortable environment in which to relax. If you want to create an amazing atmosphere, it can be done simply. Want to know the least expensive way to create the ultimate office? Good paint (I prefer deep, rich colors) and indirect, warm lighting. Turn up the heat, add some soft, gentle music and keep the dust bunnies out of the corners. People do not like to disrobe in a dirty room. Fancy that.

Do not invest thousands in art, water fountains, expensive fish tanks, and expensive electronic office gadgets. When you are big and rich, sure, add to it, but do not be foolish. I know of several people that borrowed inordinate amounts of money to create an image. Over-spending was their first mistake. How they used that money was the second. Most end up in trouble, borrow more money, and then live off of the loan money until they file for bankruptcy.

As I said earlier, it is *not* about flash. It *is* about substance. Give a great massage versus slick presentation. Your work will speak for itself.

> *Renegade Revelation:*
> *It is about the work, not the*
> *packaging.*

People that choose your services because you are cheap

will also leave because you raise your prices. I learned early on that if you are making your services about money, then your clients will as well.

In 1993, I made a massage video entitled *Massage with Confidence*. I nearly went bankrupt marketing that video and still had no success. It was priced as a $14.99 VHS videotape. I had hundreds of videos that gathered dust in my garage while I was thousands of dollars in debt.

In 1999, I decided to put my video on Amazon.com. At the time, there were 104 massage videos on Amazon, all selling for around $14.99, including a video staring Shari Belefonte, an actress/model who's dad, Harry, was a famous singer. There were also videos from Playboy, as well as other legitimate, therapeutic massage videos. Nearly all of the videos sold for around the same price. Considering my competition, I decided to list my video for $29.99. My friends thought I was nuts.

The next week, my video was on Amazon! In the sales ranking of 105 massage videos, mine was number 105. Nowhere but up, right? A few friends who had seen my video wrote reviews and posted them. All I could do was hope and wait for the sales to begin. The orders finally began trickling in until I began shipping several cases of videos to Amazon each week. Within 6-months, my video was number one! Me! Just an unknown massage therapist from Olympia, Washington, but now with a best-selling video.

Why would my video become number one? Most people understand that things of quality usually cost more. It is about *perceived* value. If you were shopping for tires and saw one set of four that cost $200 and another set of four that cost

$1,000, which would you assume were of better quality? Pricing is not just functional. Pricing positions you in the market and helps the client understand where you stand among your peers. Since most people really do not know what criteria are needed to compare therapists, most rely on price as an indicator of quality, even though the principle is ultimately flawed. You do not always get what you pay for.

> *Renegade Revelation:*
> *Don't fall into the discounting*
> *trap.*

While there are many books written on the subject of "thought-based" outcomes, "positive thinking", "putting it out there, into the universe" and even quantum physics. Regardless of what you think, the reality is that your beliefs affect your results.

While practicing on my clients during massage school, I began each massage with a short mental exercise. I told myself that I was about to give the best massage that I had ever given, that I was going to be an artist in my movement, and would allow my hands to feel what could not be seen. I was the best massage therapist in the world. Okay, not the best, but the best therapist for *that* client at *that* moment. Everyone deserved my full attention and the best massage possible.

> *Renegade Revelation:*
> *If you feel that you are not a good*
> *therapist, your hands will betray*
> *your inner voice and produce poor*
> *quality work.*
> *If you feel that you are an*
> *exceptional therapist, your hands*
> *will provide a better massage, even*
> *with the same skill set.*

It can be a challenge to work on someone who is extremely obese. When such a client came to me for treatment, I told myself that they were attractive inside and out and deserved the same caring touch as any other human being. My hands demonstrated what my mind thought.

As a school owner, I have had several applicants and students admit that they refused to work on "fat" people, those who "smell" or those who are not "clean enough." I have had men tell me they will only work on "the hot chicks." Those words, especially uttered to someone who entered this field with the desire to help others, was more than saddening to me. If I heard words like that from an applicant, they had their application fee kindly returned and along with an outright denial of acceptance into the program. If the student made such comments *after* they were enrolled, we would have "the talk" to see if a little "reeducation" would be of benefit. If they could not see the light, I helped them on a different path - a path far away from a career in massage.

Take a moment before beginning your next massage.

Let your brain have a talk with your hands. Bless the world through your amazing touch. Make a difference by allowing your hands to transmit a loving, healthy and caring touch to everyone, especially to those that appear to be unlovely.

> *Renegade Revelation:*
> *Make every massage your best yet.*

There was a famous, action-movie star who visited the health club where I worked during my early years as a massage therapist. As he walked down the main hallway, everyone either stared or looked sheepishly at him. He was trying to blend in so that he could simply use the club equipment and facilities. That was not happening. At the same time, nobody dared approach him. I could not resist.

I walked up to the actor and said, "Hi, my name is Bob Haase. I'm one of the massage therapists here at the club and I give one of the best massages in the area. You look like you could use some work and I've got a 7:00pm opening tonight." Without pause he said, "I'll take it."

"Great", I followed. "Don't be late."

Cocky? Yes. Did he show up? Yes... he was early.

If you believe in yourself, your clients are more likely to believe in you as well.

> *Renegade Revelation:*
> *Be confident in your skills.*

With memories of studying human "beef jerky" at the

Bastyr School, I was not satisfied with my knowledge of the human body. Several years before I opened my school, I called the local coroner and spoke with her about the possibility of assisting with an autopsy. At first, the coroner thought I must be some sort of freak. "Why do you want to help with an autopsy?" she quizzed.

"I'm looking to further my research of human anatomy before I open a medical massage school."

"I'll take your name and number", she said. I heard nothing for nearly a year.

Eleven months later, I received a phone call from the coroner's office. The main autopsy assistant was ill and they did not have anyone to help with the grunt work. Would I come? Hell YES! I cleared my afternoon schedule and bolted to the coroner's office.

I was instructed to "use the restroom" as soon as I arrived because I would be suited-up for the next three to four hours and would not be able to take a break until the body was sewn shut, washed clean, packaged up and put back into the refrigerator. I grinned. "Okay!" With an empty bladder, I excitedly returned to the autopsy room. I then suited up in a special, zip-up coverall, booties, special disposable over-sleeves that had to be duct taped to ensure protection, a surgery bonnet, face shield and *three* layers of gloves. I was informed that "cut bone is razor sharp" and I would be disposing of my outer gloves numerous times throughout the procedure.

The autopsy being performed was on a middle-aged man that had collapsed and died without any witnesses. That required a mandatory autopsy.

—

The very first incision, the "Y" cut, was the most disturbing. Slicing into what was otherwise normal flesh, the pathologist opened the man's chest from shoulder to sternum on both sides. He then continued down with one long cut to the pubic bone. He quickly separated the outer muscle and tissue, revealing the ribcage. Next, he opened the tool drawer to reveal the same type of long-handled pruners that my father used to trim small branches from our unwieldy trees (apparently, they cut through the bones of the ribcage just as easily.) He snipped and lifted the chest plate away, revealing the organs.

Seeing up-close and in-person, I was in awe of what I had only seen on video or in books until that point. The doctor removed the first lung and handed it to me. "Here. I need you to put this on that scale and note the exact weight, in grams, on the marker board. Make sure you say 'left lung.'" I did as he asked and then handed it back to him. He sliced it like one would a Christmas ham, in 1/2" increments. "I'm looking for anything abnormal", he explained as he diligently observed every part of the sliced organ.

This process was repeated with each organ. When he got to the liver, I was stunned at just how large it was. He said it looked normal, but wow, it was huge! As he emptied the chest and abdominal cavity of its organs, we ended up with an open thorax and abdominal cavity wrapped in a continuous, shiny, reddish lining. And there they were - the two psoas muscles - one on each side of the spine. "Those are *huge*", I said in astonishment.

"What are huge?" the doctor asked.

"The psoas muscles!"

"Those are the psoas muscles, huh? How 'bout that."

I was stunned that the doctor really did not know his muscles. I kept that thought to myself.

I was perplexed that the plastic spine and anatomy models used in schools show the psoas muscles to be fairly small, averaging less than an inch in diameter. Even my cadaver-class bodies had psoas muscles that were small because they were lacking fluids.

Autopsies made me realize that plastic anatomy models in used in schools often are crafted from what cadavers look like, not a body full of blood and fluids. The reality was that the psoas muscles were the same size as the man's wrist! The muscles were huge! It was not an anomaly either. On every subsequent autopsy, the psoas muscles were generally the same size as the person's wrists.

Ever wonder what your butt would look like if you saw it from the underside as you sat on a clear plastic chair? Perhaps slightly wider? What became clear in my research is that the quadratus lumborum is much more medial to the spine than what we usually see in books. In real "life", it is typically directly beneath the erector spinae, not lateral to it. Another common deviation is the lowest, floating ribs. The quadratus, if sufficiently in spasm, can pull those costal bones with such downward force that they are nearly touching the illiac crest. Kind of like a peace sign which is simply a broken, inverted cross.

Have you ever worked on a client who looked thin, or "skinny", but when you touched them, they felt soft and squishy? Or have you ever worked on a large person who visually appeared "fat", but when you pushed on their skin, you felt muscle tissue directly beneath the skin? The reason is something chefs refer to as "marbling."

Steaks, like top sirloin, are lean muscle covered by a layer of fat, whereas a New York steak is marbled with fat throughout the muscle tissue. The same is true with humans. Some people carry their fat predominantly on the surface of their muscle tissue while others have fat marbled throughout their muscles or hanging in large droplets off of their organs. Amazing how performing an autopsy will give you the sudden urge to start eating right. The point is, when you are working on your clients, realize that obese clients with superficial adipose tissue are going to be more difficult to treat than those with adipose marbled throughout. Again, we are all uniquely different.

With each autopsy, it became even clearer to me that there is no "normal" body. Some are missing muscles or have extra muscles. Some are missing bones or have extra bones. Others have malformed muscles while others have malformed bones... you get the picture.

> *Renegade Revelation:*
> *There is no "normal" when it*
> *comes to human anatomy and*
> *physiology.*

My autopsy experience was one of the highlights of my career and I loved every moment. Sadly, when the coroner's office learned that I cancelled hundreds of dollars in massage treatments in order to only make $50.00 for a 4-hour autopsy session, they felt guilty and stopped utilizing me as an assistant. However, they knew that I was a gallery-art photographer in my free time and asked for one final favor. They wanted to have the county's first photo documentation of a human harvest from a donor body.

That final day left me speechless. I watched as the body of a 22-year old woman, who had died in a car accident, went through 10-hours of meticulous procedures. Corneas were removed to help someone see. Skin graphs were taken to help burn victims. The heart was removed so that the valves could be used to save a life. Cervical and lumbar bones were harvested so that surgeons could give spinal injury patients a new lease on life. Arms, from shoulder to wrist, and legs, from hip to ankle, had their bones removed and replaced with two-inch dowel rods so the body looked "normal" in the casket. The bones and functioning joints would be used to help others in need. Illiums were removed so that they could later be crushed and sterilized from tissue then later utilized as "croutons" to provide a matrix from which new bone could grow.

At least fifty people would be helped because that young woman chose to give   the gift of life through donor card designation. The family would not even notice that their loved one looked any different at the time of her burial, but dozens of lives would be changed in ways that "thanks" could never express.

Revelations From My Time With The NCBTMB

In my second year as a massage therapist, I was recommended for the position of Marketing Director for the National Certification Board for Therapeutic Massage & Bodywork (NCBTMB.) I look back at that experience with both sweet and bitter memories. As with everything, there were lessons to be learned.

The first, and most direct, revelation that came of that experience was my first assignment. I was to create a brochure to be mailed to every massage therapist in the United States.

As a "marketing guy", I knew graphic design is not something you do yourself just because you have a software program. Although I had done my own graphics for years and did have some graphics training, I really needed an outside perspective. I received a bid from a well-respected, local graphics studio that wanted $2,200.00 for the job. And that was in 1993! Really? I was frustrated at the over-the-top bids I was receiving. I stopped into a Kinkos where I met a nice woman at the graphics desk. I asked her what she would charge to work with me in order to create a tri-fold flyer and she said $50.00 an hour. I was all in! We worked on the flyer for a total of three hours and I was excited about the result.

That week, I had sent a proof document to the entire board for approval. Everyone on the board looked it over and offered suggestions and corrections. I implemented the board's input, corrections were made, and a final proof was presented to the board for approval.

Eventually the entire board signed off on the flyer and the mailing was sent. If memory serves, over 60,000 flyers were mailed to the therapists throughout the United States. The mail-house sent the extra mailers to my home a week or so later and I still vividly remember opening the box of flyers. My wife, Debbie, was watching me as I proudly showed her one.

"Look! Aren't these great?" She could see the cover with big words, *"Show Your Commitment to Excelence."* I asked, "Don't they look great? We just sent these out to all of the massage therapists in the country!"

Debbie gave me a "you're not going to like what I'm about to say" smile and said, "You misspelled the word 'Excellence'."

Crap. I had every board member approve the flyer and <u>no one</u> caught that we misspelled "excellence"?! That was a huge revelation from my board experience. Be sure to have as many people as possible review your advertisements for errors! Even my daughter, Sara, at the young age of 8-years old, caught the wrong year on a brochure I had been using for some time.

> *Renegade Revelation:*
> *Get as much input and feedback as*
> *possible. Mistakes make you look*
> *like an amateur and do not cast a*
> *light of excelence on your business.*
> *Er... I mean excellence.*

Serving the board was certainly a learning experience. I will not name names, because many of those I had worked with and encountered are now nationally known, but I did find one common truth about those in power. Those at the top are often 50% image, 25% attitude and 25% content. Bottom line? Don't be intimidated by those who lead. They are probably just as concerned that they will screw-up as you are thinking that they are somehow better than you.

Renegade Revelation:
Do not be intimidated by those
who lead.

While touring massage schools throughout the country, I was able to observe students in various educational environments. It afforded the opportunity to interview both students and graduates of their programs. That experience allowed me to see and gain an understanding of something completely unexpected. I realized that a student's hours in school did not directly equate to the quality of the graduate. There was a complete disconnect between a curriculum's hours of classroom training and how good the student was at graduation.

Sure, a 2,000-hour program is bound to produce a better graduate than a 50-hour weeklong course, but most courses in the USA are averaging between 500 and 1,000 hours. I have encountered amazing therapists with incredible skills trained in 500-hour courses. I have also encountered therapists with 1,000-hours of training who cannot give a good massage or help someone get out of pain.

Recently, I had a woman in my Secrets of Deep Tissue™ seminar who had 2,000 hours of training from Canada, yet never learned deep tissue. In that same seminar, another woman, trained in Illinois, was only required to give a dozen massages during her 500-hours of training. She was head-smart, but admitted she did not have any manual skills.

My hope is that, as a profession, we are better able to both quantify the specific number of hours as well as specify the essential and necessary content that must be taught in a massage school's program. For a massage therapist to say that they have "100-hours of clinical massage" training means a lot of different things to a lot of different schools. Again, I do not want us all alike, but solid education is imperative if we are to continue to build rapport with the medical community.

> *Renegade Revelation:*
> *A therapist's hours of training*
> *does not always equate to the*
> *quality of their work.*

What I learned next I probably already understood, but was able to see demonstrated in the real world. That is, "don't believe everything you read."

Part of my job with the board was to create a video that would be used to promote national certification in massage schools throughout the USA. To shoot the raw footage we needed to interview hundreds of people in our profession. My videographer, Phil Pratt, and I embarked on a two-week adventure, flying to cities throughout the country. After interviews in Seattle, we flew from Washington to Hawaii, California, Colorado, Illinois, Texas and Florida. We had opportunity not only to interview massage therapists but also leaders in the massage profession, owners of massage schools, massage students, massage clients and even "people on the street." It truly was an awesome and eye-opening experience.

What I had previously learned from my own experience as a massage student was now confirmed. Many of our nation's schools perpetuate myth, misinformation, "old wives' tales" and mediocre curriculums. Teachers teach what they have been taught. Even if what they were taught was wrong or not based on fact.

The upside is that once an educator realizes that they are preserving bad information in their curriculums, they have the opportunity to change it. I really wish that schools would have a full time fact-checker on staff to verify the accuracy of what is being taught. Just as the medical profession increases its insights into medical truths and adjusts their courses and treatments accordingly, so too should massage schools adapt and maintain pace with the expansion of knowledge based on accurate facts.

In the early days of my school, I used to sit at the back of the room and listen to the instructors teach. My goal was to interject as little as possible so that I could gain insight about how to help my instructors improve.

One evening, a new anatomy & physiology instructor was asked a question regarding the circulatory system from a student. The instructor's answer was flat-out wrong. I had to correct the information immediately so that the students would learn the material correctly. Later, during the break, I took the teacher aside and asked her about the answer she gave. Her response was, "Well, I didn't know and I didn't want the students to think I didn't know what I was talking about so I made it up." That was the end of her A&P teaching career at my school. She could teach bodywork, but teaching science and anatomy was not her gifting. Sadly, this is a prevalent problem in massage education.

> **Renegade Revelation:**
> *If a teacher said it, it is not always true.*

There are many who believe that just because something appears in a book, it must be true. That is not the case. For example, in our school's second year, we were going to use a textbook written specifically for massage therapists. The problem was it was so full of factual mistakes that we had to send it back to the publisher. I regret not having read every word of the book before I allowed it in the school in the first place. Lesson learned. When I contacted the woman who wrote the book and self-published it, she informed me that she would not give us our money back unless we documented every mistake in the book and showed how it should be corrected. *That* was not going to happen. I told her that I would have to bill her at my "editorial consulting rate." She opted to just refund our money.

When I was a test-bank item verifier for the National Certification Exam, I was similarly stunned. On a hot summer afternoon at the Physiological Corporation in San Antonio, Texas, I sat in an air-conditioned room with a group of massage therapists who were reviewing questions that had been written by a previous group. The previous group was tasked with writing test questions including several multiple-choice answer options. My group was tasked with proposed question and answer review and approval. The basis of those questions and the "correct" answers came from a select group of approved textbooks.

My review group included massage therapists with as few as 50-hours of training (but with numerous years of experience) and upwards of 2,000-hours of massage training. Also among my group were nationally renowned educators and authors. One of those authors quickly became a little angry with me.

The moderator would read a question and then give the four potential responses, A, B, C, D, and sometimes "all" or "none" of the above. Each reviewer would give what was thought to be the right answer, out loud. If we were not all in agreement, the question was set aside for correction by a future group. At least that was how it was supposed to happen. With numerous questions, the entire group would agree on an answer except for me. I would raise my objection and say, "... and sometimes 'B'..." The moderator would dismiss my statement as being "too picky." Ignoring my objection and approving the question, the group abruptly moved on to the next question. After this happened a half-dozen times or so, the "sports massage author" sitting next to me clenched his jaw and said, "You're just being too picky!" I got up and walked out to "cool" down.

That was a mistake. Did you know it is hot, in Texas, in the summer? After walking a half-mile in 120-degree sweltering heat, I was drenched and walked back for the comfort of the building's air conditioning. Once calm, I walked back into the room and the moderator asked if I had anything I wanted to say. The room was quiet and tense. I simply said, "Either the question and approved answer is true or it is not. We can't afford to have questions on our National Exam that are 'mostly true' or true with exceptions. You all seem to believe that the content of these approved textbooks are as holy as the Bible, but you are mistaken." With that, the moderator had the group go back to take a look at the questions that I said were not good enough to use. They were thrown out.

I was now concerned about the questions that had been approved in the groups before and after ours. No test is perfect, but especially if it is perpetuating incorrect information. This brings us our *bonus* revelation: **Excellence cannot be achieved by committee.**

> *Renegade Revelation:*
> *Just because something is taught in the classroom or printed in a book, it is not necessarily true.*

Business Lessons Learned

Employees

During my 5th year in business, I had a medical massage practice adjacent to a local hospital and shared space with a local osteopathic physician. We were two separate business entities and I hired my own therapists for my side of the clinic.

At one point, I had hired a woman who had known me since childhood, as well as one of her friends. Things went really well for the first few months until they both found themselves in a discussion with several other massage therapists. The topic was compensation and how their respective employers were paying each of them. In the course of that discussion, my two employees learned that the other therapists were getting paid a higher percentage of the treatment fee than I was paying them. They were more than upset by that news.

The next day, both employees sat me down for a heart-to-heart talk. They told me of their discussion with the other therapists regarding the differences in pay structures. I was slightly agitated and told them that I was paying them what we had agreed upon, which we had all decided was fair compensation. I made it clear that their employment contracts specifically stated that they were not to disclose my company's policies with outsiders. I went on to explain how they only had to show up and make money. I paid for everything... pagers (yes, we used pagers back in the day), linens, oils and medical billing. I provided advertising, business cards and was responsible for bringing every client, whom they were treating, through the door. They left the meeting a little frustrated and I mistakenly thought that was the end of the discussion.

The woman, who I had known since childhood, confronted me two weeks later. She informed me that she had spoken with additional therapists and employers regarding her compensation package. She felt that I "needed to know" I was not paying them fairly. I asked her if she understood me when I had told her that if she were to again divulge internal policies to our competition that she would be let go. She admitted that she understood and then handed me her resignation. The contempt in her eyes kept me from trying to retain her as an employee. It was clear that more discussion would not change anything.

The remaining therapist seemed content that she still had a job, but confronted me again. Her new strategy was to ask for "a raise."

"You only pay me 55% of the massage fee. My friends make 70% and I think I deserve a raise."

I looked at her, trying to conceal my disbelief. I explained, "I pay you more than the other employers pay. Do you realize that?" She emphasized that I was not paying a "high enough *percentage*."

I knew I needed to speak clearly and be succinct. "Look, my clinic charges $100.00 per hour, so you make $55.00. Your friends make 70% of their employer's $60.00 fee, earning them $42.00 per hour. You are making more than every employed therapist in town." She still did not get it.

"But, you aren't paying me a high enough percentage! I want a raise!", she said emphatically.

That was it. I realized I had to get the point across with a little more clarity. "Okay, you're right", I sighed. "You really should get a higher percentage than what I am paying you. So, from now on, I am going to give you 90% of the massage fee."

"REALLY?!", she asked with a big smile.

"Yep. Oh, but so you know, I am lowering my fees to just $1.00 per massage. You'll make 90-cents."

She was upset. "That's not fair!"

It was at that point that I let my employee go. The bottom line is, never negotiate percentages of gross fees with employees. What I learned from that experience was to ask a new employee how much they felt was fair for me to pay them on an hourly basis. For example, let us say that a new employee said she wanted to be paid $40.00 per 50-minute session. I would say, "Okay, so you feel that being paid $40.00 an hour is fair. Do you think it is fair for me to add, to what I pay you, an additional sum to run my business and keep the clients coming in the door?"

The employee would always say yes. In the future, raises were just that, raises. If they wanted more and I felt they deserved it, any future increase would be independent of the amount that I charged the client. It was a win-win strategy and everyone was ultimately happy.

> *Renegade Revelation:*
> *NEVER pay employees a*
> *percentage of the massage fee.*

I realized that I could not afford to have employees working for me that did not understand what makes a business work. In the long run, if employees do not grasp the basics of how successful businesses operate, they can ultimately become a detriment to the business. Also, if employees get the impression that employment is a right of entitlement and they are "owed" a job, they truly will have no concern for the success of their employer. They can ultimately bankrupt the company and simply move on to the next job.

If employees *expect* their employers to care about their best interests, they too should have their employer's best interests in mind. In other words, do not chew on the hand that feeds you. Both need to be invested in the other's well being. It is a symbiotic relationship. Cory Garnaas, my best friend and CPA, has said repeatedly over the years, "*Nobody cares about your business as much as you. Nobody.* "

Here is the takeaway... You do not need to create business students. You *do* need to develop relationships with your employees and demonstrate that you care about their individual success, as well as show them how they benefit by participating in your business' success.

Have you ever heard the story of the scorpion and the frog? In short, the frog gave the scorpion a ride across the river on its back. The scorpion gave the frog a fatal sting before they reached the other side. As the frog was dying and both were sinking, the frog asked "Why?"

"It's my nature", the scorpion replied.

How does this fit? If the employee hurts the company as a result of their actions, both the company and employee fail. They must both work together in order to achieve long-term success, by mutually respecting each other. Both must be vested in contributing to the success of the other.

In my early years as an employer, my percentage-based employees and independent contractors would call in the morning to inquire about what their schedule looked like for the day. Since I did not pay them a wage in between massages, they felt the liberty to come and go as they pleased. This included canceling out their availability if there was a block of time when they did not have clients scheduled. Invariably, a client would call and ask for an appointment and I would have to say, "I'm sorry, I don't have any openings today." This expensive habit was ultimately my fault because I was unwilling to pay them to sit around between massages appointments.

Eventually, I sat down and figured out how much my employees averaged per hour, during an 8-hour work shift. I then hired therapists to work specific shifts and paid them that hourly amount whether they were massaging, answering calls, filing, making coffee, or sterilizing equipment. It was my job to keep them busy. With a therapist always available, my income increased and my stress levels decreased.

> *Renegade Revelation:*
> *Independent contractors may save*
> *you in taxes, but you will likely*
> *lose out on potential income and*
> *profit in the long run.*

Employees are not always honest. Sad to say, but it is

true. Whether it is taking a 39-cent ballpoint pen home in a shirt pocket, or lying about their hours, it happens. Let me share two experiences in which my employees committed "time" theft...

The first time I was "robbed at pen-point" was by a woman who I had hired through a temp agency. She seemed nice and got her work done. I later found out that she and her husband were having financial difficulties.

One afternoon, I noticed that she had signed her timesheet after returning from lunch. She wrote down "12:45pm." The trouble was, I distinctly remember her getting back at 1:00pm. Over the next two days I observed that she signed in on her timesheet 15-minutes before she actually arrived as well as 15-minutes later than she actually left. She was stealing 15-minutes at the start of her day, 15-minutes before lunch, 15-minutes after lunch, and 15-minutes at the end of the day! She stole *one whole hour* every day. I called the employment agency that evening, and arranged for a new temp to begin the next morning. Lesson learned.

The second time an employee cheated on a timesheet, it amounted to the largest theft in my company's history. As my school grew larger, it was time to hire a "Dean of Students." After numerous interviews, we decided to hire a nice, middle-aged, divorced woman with a daughter in college.

She requested an hourly wage near the high end of what I was willing to pay and she insisted that she was worth every penny. "I don't like salaried positions", she clarified. "It's too easy for the employer to take advantage of the employee." That statement would soon prove ironic.

She was full of spunk and always made sure I knew she

was "busy" with multiple projects throughout her daily workload. At the end of her first pay cycle, my campus manager forwarded the employee's timesheets. The bulk of the timesheets were for our numerous teachers, while the others were administrative positions, which included the Dean of Students.

To clarify, the pay cycle was from the 1st through the 15th of the month. There are an average of 4.33 weeks in a month, based on a 40-hour workweek. The average full- time employee would have worked about 86.67 hours in that semi-monthly pay period. When I looked at her time sheet, it had **196**-hours as her *total* time. I looked at it again.

She claimed 109-hours of overtime. My heart raced.

I immediately called my campus manager and asked her to explain why our new employee had worked so many hours. She did not know. She said she would call her and get back to me. The Dean of Students explained to my campus manager that she had "lots to do in order to organize the office and put out fires from all of the issues that weren't handled" prior to her arrival. She also had to "take a lot of work home."

Immediately, I changed our company's employee manual to include a paragraph that stated "no overtime was allowed unless previously approved by the management in writing."

The following pay period arrived. She claimed "184-hours" of work which amounted to 98-hours of overtime. I called my campus manager and asked the same question as before, with slightly increased color in my language. What was her excuse this time? More "take-home work" and hours that we could not verify.

She was warned, in writing, that she had broken school policy and it could *not* happen again. I instructed my campus manager to look at the time sheets – daily - to ensure it would not happen again. Even with my clear instruction, it happened again.

The next pay period arrived. Sure enough, 182-hours were listed. I made three phone calls. The first was to my campus manager to find out why she had not kept a daily eye on the time sheet. She responded that the Dean never entered her hours until after the pay period was over. Hmm.

The second call was to my attorney. He said, "If she says she worked the hours, you must pay her - even if it is fraudulent. You can pay her, or you can pay her and then fire her. Either way, you must pay her."

Our conversation about employee behavior was enlightening that day. For example, if a postal worker signs in, goes "postal", kills everyone, and signs out, then the postal service must pay him - even if he did not do his job. They can pay him, or they can pay him and then fire him. Either way, he is getting paid. *Wow!*

My third call was to the Dean. I told her that she had obviously not worked 80-90 hour workweeks, but had padded her hours. "You are stealing from me, and that is unconscionable." She gave the excuse that she had a daughter in college and that she needed the money.

The bottom line is, as a business owner, you must keep an eye on your business. That means *daily*. Know what is happening and watch out for your investment. Remember, nobody cares about your business as much as you do.

> *Renegade Revelation:*
> *Employees have been known to lie,*
> *cheat and steal.*

A few months after the Dean of Students incident, my campus manager left the school. Her departure left a void. Although I handled her responsibilities for a short time, I sought someone else to do the job. Truthfully, managing a school was not my heart's desire.

A woman dropped by the school one afternoon. She had a lot of teaching experience with my largest competitor - a school several times the size of mine. Although currently employed by the other school, she told me that she would quit if I hired her because she wanted to live in Olympia. This all sounded reasonable to me.

To call the school for a reference was not an option because it would tip them off to her seeking employment elsewhere. I had to settle for calling one of her colleagues. This was not my usual method of operation, but I sympathized with her situation, so it would have to do. She was confident, well spoken and seemed to be a good fit for our school, so I hired her.

Two weeks after she joined the staff, she told me that she would love to take on the role of campus manager and would do so for a reasonable wage. She assured me that it would give me the freedom to relax and do what I do best. I was not in the mood to let the opportunity pass and promptly promoted her.

A week later, she informed me that she was a lesbian. I

wondered why she felt it necessary to tell me that. I have never felt the urge to tell employers for whom I have worked that I was a heterosexual, so why would she share this information? She knew that if I fired her after she revealed her sexual preference, she could potentially have a case against me for unlawful dismissal. You cannot fire employees because they are gay. Ever. It really did not matter because I had no plans to fire her.

A week later, she had a "confession" to make. Her life-partner was the president and director of the school she had recently left. Nice. My campus manager was sharing pillow talk about the inner workings of my company with the president of my competition. What could possibly go wrong?! I did not sleep well that night.

This might sound obvious, but my competition really was not happy that my school existed. Based on geography, my school was a much closer and more economical option for many of the students who would have otherwise gone to their school. I was costing them money. I also produced exceptional graduates and word had gotten out that their students did not have the level of skills that mine did. I was costing them money and their reputation as well.

My campus manager promised that she would never talk about my school to her partner or reveal inside information. Ever.

Over the next few weeks, my employees had started to act differently. They seemed stressed. Some would not look me in the eye. One teacher finally came to me and said, "I can't do this. I can't work for her any longer. She is a tyrant and I'm tired of being threatened. I quit."

Even after I smoothed things over with my teacher and confronted the campus manager, things felt uncomfortable between the two of them. "It was a misunderstanding", she insisted.

Several days later I observed the campus manager quickly close her office door as she saw me enter the school. Seconds later, her personal phone line lit-up as she placed an outside call. She had never before closed her office door to use the phone. Two days later, she again closed the door to make a call. My gut told me that something was wrong. I picked up my phone and hit a secret sequence of numbers that allowed me to listen in on her call.

Now, before you gasp at my actions, know that every employee signed our employee handbook that states they understood our policies. One of those policies in particular stated that nothing was private in the school administrative offices. We reserved the right to monitor all communications that took place at the school including email, web browsing and telephone calls. Did I actually monitor those communications? No. I had more important things to worry about - at least until that particular day.

While I listened to the call, I heard the campus manager's voice talking with her partner. They used low tones, as if trying to avoid being overheard. My fears were realized. She was telling her partner about things that were taking place at my school and strategies that we were using to increase student enrollments. My hair stood up on the back of my neck.

I called our receptionist, at the front desk and asked her to bring me the school's phone bills for the past two months.

After I poured over those bills, it became clear that the campus manager had made and received literally hundreds of calls to and from my competition's phone number. Dozens of hours of phone time in just two months. I listened in again and heard more of the same. It was apparent that my company was under surveillance. While this was not the stuff of spy novels, I certainly had a "mole" that seemed to be working with the competition and determined to damage my company. That afternoon, I attempted to interview the other teachers and staff, but each seemed leery to talk with me. "I don't want to lose my job", was the response that several gave when I called them. Things were worse than I thought.

I immediately started preparations to put a new campus manager in place. He was an ex-navy officer and graduate of my school. He literally knew how to turn a ship around and was set to begin at 5:00 pm that Friday. My meeting with the current campus manager was set for 4:00 pm. The transition was smooth, but until her departure, I really had no idea of how bad things really were.

Apparently, my competition was more upset with our small school than I realized. They set out to steal my curriculum and destroy the vocational school that I had worked so hard to painstakingly build from the ground up. The outgoing campus manager had informed the employees that they would be fired if they said anything about how things were being run. Sadly, the poor receptionist was told to shred two, full years of student records and if she did not, or if she told anyone, she would be fired.

There was more – *a lot* more. But my point is this: Jealous people will try to destroy you. Whether with gossip, slander or outright devious actions, these people do not want to see you succeed. Prepare for the worst, but expect the best.

I have always treated my employees well and tried to create a good working environment. Those same employees whom you try to treat well will, on occasion, do their best to hurt you. Again, be prepared.

> *Renegade Revelation:*
> *Your competition does not have*
> *your best interests in mind.*

There are a range of personalities which you will encounter as an employer ranging from the "OMG, everything is out of control" to the "I'm done, what else can I do?" employee. I'll keep this section short since this is not a book on personality types and testing, but there have been several types of employees that I have commonly encountered as a business owner and each can affect your business in unexpected ways:

1.   <u>The type that wants your job</u>. They want to learn all they can and improve on it. Their appetite for growth, potential and success is insatiable. They might make you money in the short run, but they will not be there long and will likely leave a mess in the wake of their departure. Employ with caution.

2.   <u>The type that just wants to collect a paycheck</u>. They are what I call the "sloths" of the office who act busy enough not to get fired, but actually produce as little as possible. They create a lot of

busywork while being watched, but are usually cruising the internet when you are not watching.

3.	<u>The type that needs to convince you that they are indispensable to insure they keep their job</u>. This is similar to the last type, but more drama-based. They tend to have messy desks and act as though they have far too much work to do, but because they are a trooper, they will persevere. They eat your time and are usually giving off an "I'm so exhausted because I'm working so hard for you mentality.

4.	<u>The person who has a good work ethic and enjoys doing a good job</u>. They can usually take two hours to do the amount of work that a "drama" employee can do in a full day. If they are exceptional, they will find other ways to fill their day making the business a better place to work or come up with ideas to keep themselves busy on their own. Pay this type of employee more than they expect. They are gold.

5.	<u>The person who is always negative.</u> Do not let office politics get a foothold on robbing employees of their joy. If they have a complaint about the work place, they need to talk to the manager, not their fellow employees. The same holds true for you as the manager or owner. Especially if you have issues that you are working through outside of the office, never discuss them inside the confines of the work environment. Talk to a counselor or mental health therapist if you must, but do not spill the details of your life to your employees or open your ears to the gossip and emotional dumping that employees hope you will entertain. It makes for an unhealthy work environment. If they need a counselor, give them a few, good names.

Keep in mind that there are numerous employee types. If you are going to hire someone, it is worth learning more about whom and how to properly hire. Time well spent in the hiring process saves an incredible amount of time and money later.

To me, what is most important when hiring an employee is to ascertain what motivates an applicant. Take the time to figure this out because all employees are not alike. Some know exactly what motivates them. Some do not have a clue. Things that motivate employees may include:

- Stability
- Opportunity
- Danger
- Autonomy
- Being part of a group
- Opportunity to make a lot of money yet incur some of the risk
- A steady paycheck that is consistent in amount and frequency
- A chance to have a creative outlet

Understanding what motivates them will help insure you are providing them what they need to feel safe so they can do their best for you, allowing you to provide them the best job that they have ever had.

While many employers have the "they need me more than I need them" philosophy, they are wrong. A good employee can make or break a company. Their decisions can drive the company into excellence and prosperity, or bring it down in flames and destruction. Your decision to truly respect, value and motivate your employees will reap lasting rewards for your company as well as decreased stress for you.

> *Renegade Revelation:*
> *Read a book about common*
> *personality types of employees.*

If you write another human being a paycheck and they are not an equal partner in your business, they are not your friend. Do not confuse what feels like friendship as actual friendship. Do not hang out together. Do not party together. Do not t tell them about your marital troubles and especially do not tell them about your company's financial troubles.

I am not saying that familiarity with an employee will always go wrong. However, I can say that when you treat employees like friends it is the foundation for boundary confusion that leads to even bigger problems later.

> *Renegade Revelation:*
> *Employees are not your friends.*

When hiring an employee, I have found it is always best to require a 90-day probation period. What they say in their interview and how they actually perform versus what a reference inferred are often two, or even three, very different things. Contracts will bind you to a situation. In order to be released from a contract, you may have to pay dearly. That said, letters of clarification are important for subcontractors as well as employees. Simple language is key. Be sure to include what they will do and what their responsibilities are, as well as what you will do and what you will provide. Clarify pay, benefits, leave, vacations, etc. Make sure you include the phrase, "This is an 'at will' agreement." See your business attorney for more information. Trust me, spending a few dollars with your attorney now will save you much more later.

It is an important part of your hiring process - for both employees and subcontractors - that you have them read and sign your employee handbook and/or company policy manual. Keep a signed copy in their file and make sure that whenever you change your policies that you get a new signature.

Posting important policies is also important. You never want an "I had no idea!" comment coming from your employees. Cover policies in meetings and make sure that everyone knows them and understands what you expect in terms of conduct. You cannot have a successful massage clinic if you have employees breaking your policies.

Renegade Revelation:
Employee contracts are a bad idea.

Unless you plan to create a large corporation devoid of your presence, partnerships are a bad idea. Cory Garnaas and I were having a drink one night, talking about the future of my company. Great ideas were flying everywhere. We were honing the details of what would make my new business successful. I asked Cory if I should have business partners. Cory sat his drink down on the bar, looked me in the eye and, without missing a beat, said: "Bob... partnerships are like marriages, but without any sex." Take on employees, not partners.

I know of a doctor in town that decided to take on two partners. To entice the other doctors to join his practice, he gave them each a stake on the company. Two months later, the other two doctors held 66% of the partnership combined and voted the original doctor out of the business. Be forewarned.

> *Renegade Revelation:*
> *Avoid "silent partners" or*
> *investors in your company.*

There is no need to sell mousetraps in a city that does not have mice. If you are a massage therapist opening a business amongst fifty other therapists, hanging a sign out your window with the word "Massage" on it will doom you to failure. Unless you have a client base already, make sure you create a market niche that makes you unique in a sea of blandness. Differentiation is mandatory for success.

A friend of mine attended an Assemblies of God Bible college to become a pastor. When he graduated, he spent some time at a church out of state. Then he felt that he was supposed to start a church in the same town where his parents lived. I suspect it was more about convenience versus calling, but that is not my judgment to make. As a friend, however, I get to ask the tough questions of my friends, as they do with me.

I do not intend to start a religious debate here, but the story is important, so I will keep this short.

Some large, religious organizations want to build, or "plant" churches in communities that do not have the funds to do so themselves. These benevolent organizations will do so because there is a need and they feel that the community will suffer without their generosity. In other words, they know it will cost money to have a church there, but the purpose outweighs the potential financial loss the organization will likely incur.

Other religious organizations require local churches to build their own buildings. They then charge that church what would be considered a "franchise fee" of sorts, with a percentage of the church offerings and donations going back to the organization. Much like, a local catholic church ultimately sends money to Vatican City.

When my friend decided to build a church in a rural Northwest town, I asked him the population of the city. At the time, about 25-years ago, the population was around 6,000. Then I asked how many churches were already in the small community. "About 40 or so", was his reply.

I said, "There are more than two-times the number of churches in your town than there are restaurants. Since people eat out more than they go to church, and people typically only attend one church rather than multiple churches each week, do you really feel there is a need for *one more* church in your town?" He had not given it much thought. Unless he was starting a new religion, the community had no need for yet another church. The population was already having their needs met by the existing churches. Yes, a church is a business, with bills, expenses and payroll - especially when it is not being funded by a philanthropic organization. He opened his church, only to close its doors a year later. There may have been potential church members in the community, but there was no need for an additional church.

So how does the story of starting a church apply to the massage therapist? Simple. You need to determine need and potential. If I were to consider opening a massage office or clinic in your town, I would ask a number of questions, such as:

- What is the population of your town?
- What is the geographic location? (e.g.: Is it a town from, or to, which people commute, thereby increasing or decreasing the population during business hours)
- How many massage therapists are already established in your town?
- What percentage of the population gets regular massage or bodywork?
- In what kind of bodywork do you specialize?
- How many in your town are already providing your specific type of bodywork?

Once you know the potential and details about your true competition, you can make a better judgment on how to proceed. In a recent national study by the American Massage Therapy Association, they found:

- There was an 83% increase in massage therapists

nationally from 1998 to 2008, totaling 288,546 in the field, give or take.

- In 2009, 18% of men received massage compared to 26% of women.
- Women receive massage twice as often as men.
- Baby Boomers (ages 55-64) have doubled their massage use over the past decade and those over 65 have tripled their use.
- By contrast, younger consumers (18-34) have reduced their consumption of massage (The economy has likely had an impact since this group has less disposable income).
- Only 10% of households making under $35,000 annually get massage, but 43% of households making over $100,000 a year get massage by comparison.
- In 2011, 18% of Americans received a massage in the previous year; 31% in the previous 5-years.
- 32% of consumers get massage to "pamper" themselves.
- 32% of consumers get massage for medical reasons on average (45% of males receive massage for medical reasons.)
- 41% of those 55-65 years of age get massage for medical reasons.
- 86% of the US population believes that massage therapy can be a beneficial and effective way to reduce pain.
- 25% of patients between 35 and 44 years of age spoke with their physician about massage. Of those that spoke to their physicians about massage, 52% of the

doctors recommended massage.

- 40% of the population considers massage therapy to manage stress.
- 39% of women that receive massage do so to manage stress as opposed to 22% of males

So how do you use this information to make decisions about opening or altering a massage practice? You can make some extrapolations just by reading over the data. For example, if you are in a town with a population of 50,000, that means roughly 9,000 people may be receiving massage this year. Some may receive on a weekly basis and others only once. But then again, frequency depends on how good a massage is and if the therapist is educating the client.

Back when I was in college, my buddies would compare any purchase to "pizza and beer" economics. If I were going to buy a new piece of audio equipment, they would say, "DUDE! Instead of that, you could buy 25-pizzas and 10-racks of beer!" Massage is like that. People do not necessarily *need* massage to survive or live their lives. However, if the massage is good, they will forego the "pizza and beer." If the massage is not so good in their area, they have a feast and self-medicate their pain away. Percentages of the population receiving massage are directly affected by the therapists in a given market or geographical region.

With this simple math, you can make a decision as to whether there is room for another therapist based on the current number of therapists offering massage. If you are an injury treatment/medical massage-focused therapist working with adults of retirement age and most of the other therapists in town are spa or relaxation therapists, it would not matter how many therapists there were... there is a need for *your* services.

I remember driving down the road on my way to lunch with a doctor buddy of mine and I saw yet another teriyaki restaurant. *Another* one! Our side of town already had 8 of them. How did they market themselves? They put out a white banner with red letters that read: "Teriyaki." The depth of advertising creativity astonished me. There was one car in the parking lot at the noon hour. If all of the Teriyaki restaurants were full at lunchtime, the necessity of a new restaurant would make sense. It would even make sense if they were providing something that was different and new, but they were not. They were just offering the same as the rest in an already saturated market. Know your customer. Most business owners create a product or service that they think the public wants and then try to market it. Wrong approach. Find out what the public wants and then fill that need better than anyone else. Have you asked your clients about what they want? What would they like to have available if they could create the ultimate massage office/clinic? Remember, they may be happy because they already like what you offer and that is why they utilize your services.

If your practice is not as busy as you would have hoped, you may be able to bring in additional clients by making some changes. Start asking people their opinions. Send out surveys and get input from as many people as you can. You may be able to make some simple adjustments to your business and the services that it offers which will make your clinic more successful and more desirable than your competition.

Just remember this... there is always a need for something that meets a need that is not being currently met. Period. Position yourself by being unique and then get the word out that you are filling their need exceptionally well.

> *Renegade Revelation:*
> *The reason you create a new*
> *business should be to fill an*
> *unfulfilled need within the*
> *community.*

Additional Business Revelations

From all my years in business, I have gleaned a lot of practical wisdom that can help you grow as a successful massage therapist and businessperson. In addition to the many businesses with whom I have coached and consulted, I have helped hundreds of massage therapists over the years. I have used my own experiences as well as personal research to arrive at my conclusions. While this is not a business book, per se, it is important to realize that just because you are a good therapist it does not guarantee that you will be a successful one. Here are some random thoughts that will help guide you:

1. The biggest mistake that causes unnecessary stress is trying to do too many things at once. It is better to do one thing well than five things with mediocrity. If you cannot do something well, hire it out. Not a graphic designer? Hire it out. Not good at taxes? Hire a CPA. Not an organized person? Hire someone to do your cleaning or someone to help create an office area that makes sense with good workflow. Do what you do best. Keep in mind that when you are not being tied-up with the daily minutia, you have the time to think, plan and achieve excellence in your company. Success takes planning and forethought.

2. Do not *spend* a dollar to *save* 30-cents. I chuckle every time I hear a therapist say, "I need to buy some stuff for my business so I do not have to pay as much in taxes." Seriously? This is not high-stakes money with offshore accounts in the Cayman Islands (although, feel free to open an account there while on my next continuing

education cruise in the Caribbean.) This is simple math. If you have $30,000 in profit, you have to spend your profit on business expenses to pay less in taxes. That means you spend the money first, and then spend less on taxes. If you are in the 28% tax bracket, then you save 28-cents every time you spend a dollar of your profit. That is foolish. Spending one dollar to make 28-cents sounds like a con game, but business people unwittingly burn their money every day without realizing that paying tax means you have made a profit. That is a good thing. See your local CPA for details.

3. Living off of borrowed money is like a farmer using his seed for the next year's crops as a breakfast cereal. A farmer should eat from the *excess* of his crops. He should not eat the seed that he needs to plan for another harvest. If you borrow money to start your business, use that money for your business and not to live on.

4. Have a clear and concise purpose, objective and mission statement written. Why? You will not know when you have arrived if you do not know where you are going. An objective and mission statement are always part of a good business plan. I offer a free, simplified business plan for therapists to download on my haasemyotherapy.com website. If you truly want to succeed while working for yourself, it is important to understand this type of planning. Like an old tee-shirt I bought in Hawaii years ago procalims, "The un-aimed arrow never misses." Sage wisdom.

5. Money is a tool, not a goal. Why is this business advice?

Good question. How you view money and how you let money affect you can have long-reaching consequences into the very fabric of your business and into your personal life.

Success is not how much money you have, but what you do with that money. Money should never be your goal. There will never be enough. If you desire to make $10,000.00 a month, what do you do when you reach that? Make $15,000.00 a month? You are chasing the end of a rainbow. However, if you have specific goals for your life, money is then merely a means to attain that goal.

As I read the book, *The 4-Hour Workweek*, by Timothy Ferriss, this concept was made even clearer to me. In essence, the author was saying that Americans work their whole lives to save enough money so that they can relax and travel. Why do we wait until we are old and our bodies betray us before we finally do what we have dreamed of all our lives? Why not do it now instead? We need to learn to change how we live while living on less. More importantly, to make money without working so hard for it so that we have the health and free time to travel. Tim tells you how to automate your income and then travel for pennies on the dollar. It is a great book and a fun read. Buy it. When you are done with that, you will also enjoy his book, *The 4-Hour Body*, especially as a health practitioner.

The bottom line is this: If you want a new boat, ask yourself "why?" Is the boat really what you want? The boat should not be the goal. Rather, look at what that boat does for you or what it allows you to do, which is to go out on the open water and have fun while doing it. Are there other ways to achieve that same outcome which will not require wheelbarrow loads of money and hours of maintenance that will rob you of your valuable free time? When you write out your goals, look at outcomes versus the means to get there. It is about the *experiences* on the water, not a boat with a money-guzzling motor. If you change your perspective, you will have more options in order to attain your goals, which may take you on an even more amazing journey.

6. Working 90-hours a week to provide for a family will usually become 90-hours a week working to pay child support, spousal maintenance and alimony. I do not mean to sound like a fatalist. I have personally come to realize that except for providing for the basic needs of your family - like food and shelter - your work is not nearly as important as your family. Nothing is worse than losing them because your priorities have spun out of balance. When your loved ones start feeling that your work is more important than everything else in your life, especially them, the consequences may not be what you had hoped. Live simpler and have the time to love and build relationships with those that you love rather than work so long and hard that the house is

empty when you get home. Trust me, I know this all too well.

7.   Do not deal with your massage linens and laundry. Early in my career, I realized that I spent a lot of time and frustration cleaning linens for my thriving massage clinic. Your residential washing machine can never compete with a commercial machine that basically boils the sheets and strips every impurity and evil out of them. It is like a professional exorcism of filth! Geez, you can eat off of the sheets when the professionals are finished with them. Sterile, white and amazingly clean, and all you have to do is open the package. Renting a linen service's sheets will always be the least time-consuming option.

It does not stop with sheets. Hire out everything that does not bring you joy... windows, janitorial, billing, etc. You make more money per hour than the professionals who can take those other tasks off of your hands. Give yourself the extra time in your day - time to think, plan, market and massage. It is the small stuff that will keep you from getting the big stuff done.

You may be thinking that you cannot afford a linen service or billing service. What I can tell you is this: *Everything* is negotiable. Everything. I negotiated with my linen service, dropping the price by 25%. Even your billing service will negotiate. Better yet, offering someone extra work at a great hourly wage to use your computer and software at your office, ultimately saving significantly.

8.   Give more than is expected. I am not saying that you should add bonus time to the end of a 60-minute massage. Adding time to a massage without first discussing it with your client is not a gift if that unexpected "bonus" time makes a parent late to pick-up their children from daycare or makes a businessperson late for a meeting. What I do mean is go beyond normal expectations. Whether it is a free bottle of water or an article that you clipped from a magazine which has to do with their profession; show your client that you care and that they are not just another client filling your schedule.

9.   You are not a commodity, so do not advertise yourself as one. Have you ever bought sugar in a grocery store? Do you care if it is house brand or another? Sugar is sugar, right? It comes in 1 lb, 5 lb, 10 lb and 25 lb bags. How much does it cost per pound? The price-per-pound is listed right there on the shelf. The customer looks at the commodity and the price and then buys what makes the most sense. With sugar, there is usually a "house brand" that the grocery store sells with their chain's own label, and one higher-level brand. The consumer buys the "cheap one" or the "good one." If there were dozens of different brands, the consumer would likely switch from "cheap or good" to becoming unsure about what to buy and then compare based on price   alone.

With massage therapy, there may be many massage therapists in a given city from which to choose. Most therapists worry and think that price must be what the consumer uses to choose a therapist. Do you believe that? If you do, it becomes the truth. The fact is, consumers do not usually know what questions to ask in order to decide if they value and want your services.

Years ago when I shared space with the osteopathic physician, my clinic was called Bodymechanics Myotherapy & Massage. My business name started with a "B", so I received a lot of calls from people working their way through the phone book asking, "How much do you charge for a one-hour massage?" I was the most expensive massage therapist in town. When I would tell them my price, they would say, "Okay, thanks", and hang up. I grew tired of the price-shopping mentality.

Due to a frustrating phone call with an insurance company one, August day, I was not in the best of moods and I really should not have answered the phone when it rang, but I did. The conversation went like this:

Me: "Thanks for calling Bodymechanics, this is Robert."

Potential client: "Uh, how much do you charge for a one-hour massage?"

Me: "You buy cars like that?"

Potential client: "Uh, what??"

Me: "Do you buy cars like that?"

Potential client: "I'm confused. What do you mean?"

Me: "Do you call a car dealership and ask 'What do you charge for a car?' Do you care if it is a Cadilac, Porsche, Yugo, or Camry?"

Potential client: "Uh..."

Me: "I'm sorry. What do you need specifically? What are you needing me to work on?"

Potential client: "Oh, I have a headache and want to feel better."

Me: "So, what you are asking is how much do I charge to get rid of your headache?"

Potential client: "Yes."

Me: "Okay. Look, an hour-long massage treatment for a headache is way too much. Also, I charge a lot for what I do. All you need is a half-hour treatment, at most, for what you are dealing with. And that costs $50.00, but if I don't give you relief, I won't charge you a penny. Now how much do I cost?"

Potential client: "Do you have an opening at 3'o'clock?"

I took the focus off of *cost* and onto the *benefit*. Never make what you do about money. There is no other therapist that offers the same exact skill set or experience. Do not price your massage like sugar in a grocery store. You need to remove your prices from your brochures. It is not about money. When people ask what I charge? I say, "A lot. I'm really expensive." It gets them curious and they usually come to see me for treatment. And yes, this applies to those of you who think that people in your small community cannot afford what you charge, but that is another discussion addressed in my marketing seminar. (See www.haasemyotherapy.com for details.)

10.   You have one chance for a first-impression.
- Be careful about your level of professionalism with your voicemail message and choose professional vs. funny
- Provide creative, quality content on your website and have someone else proofread it
- Dress well and professionally in public
- Do not get drunk in public
- Keep your office clean
- Do not have pets roaming about your office
- Return phone calls quickly

You get my point...

11.   Bigger does not usually mean better in business. My attorney, Steve Bean, once told me about his classmate

in law school who has a large legal practice in downtown Seattle with over 100 attorneys. The practice is located in a high-rise office building and has a great deal of notoriety, prestige and social status. Steve said, "Bob, in my office I have two attorneys and a few legal assistants and secretaries. At the end of the year, after paying bills and taxes, then splitting the profit with my partner, my friend in Seattle makes *the same* amount of money as I do. Don't get big, just be excellent at what you do." It is true. Aspirations of being big do not always equate to financial success or monetary gain, but becoming big will nearly always give you larger headaches.

12. The type of advertising that worked last year may not work again this year. Do not become complacent in your business. When I started my massage school, I spent $10,000.00 in advertising on Mixx96 FM radio, $10,000.00 on billboards and $5,000.00 in display ads in the local newspaper. If I were to start a school today, those same dollars, in the same media, would lead to definite failure.

Starting a new business and educating a public that had no idea my business, existed forced me not only to know my market, but also which media would most likely reach my target market. The answer to "which one" changes constantly. I am sure that you are aware TV Guide magazine has lost a significant portion of the advertising market share, just like "yellow page" advertising has lost it's effectiveness. Do you read *the*

Saturday Evening Post like your grandparents or great-grandparents? Probably not. Times change. You need to adapt your marketing strategies as well so that you do not waste your money and miss your target market.

13. Do not put all of your eggs in one basket. When you consider types of clientele, advertising media or revenue streams, relying on one single source is a huge mistake. Some examples:

- If you are running your clinic with 100% of your referrals coming from just one specific physician or from a medical insurance preferred provider agreement, you are likely setting yourself up for trouble. Should the doctor change his mind and start referring to someone else, your income may screech to a halt. Or, if you are no longer able to be a provider for the insurance company, your revenue stream ends. Always make sure you have multiple revenue streams.

- If you put all of your advertising dollars into one specific media, or worse yet, into a large, one-time advertisement, your odds of success are poor at best. With advertising, you need to have "saturation" before worrying about "reach." In other words, it is better to put a smaller advertisement in a magazine numerous times on a regular basis than one large advertisement once. People need repetition to finally realize, "Oh yeah, that looks familiar, I've seen that before, I should call them." One large ad will not do that for you.

Think of saturation and reach like watering a field of grass during the dryness of summer. The *potential* for growth is good if the grass receives enough moisture. If you have 4-acres of grass, you can either water the entire 4-acres with 1/4" of water, or you can water 1-acre with 1" of water. Cover a large area with too little water and you will get poor results. Cover a smaller area (reach) with more water to saturate the roots (saturation) and you will have great results.

Years ago, when I produced my video, *Massage with Confidence*, I decided to put a ¾-page advertisement in *TV Guide Magazine*. At the time, that was the best way to find out what was on the television. It was also when the shows *Friends* and *Seinfeld* were strong in the ratings on Thursday nights. I just "knew" that if I put one, huge, expensive advertisement in the TV guide in the Thursday night line-up with right-hand placement that was directed at the entire west coast market of 2,600,000 readers, I could not lose. If just 1% bought my video, I would be rich!

I borrowed $7,500 from a credit card and ran my single, ¾-page advertisement. What I did not count on was that there would literally be dozens of wildfires and forest fires throughout all of California and parts of Oregon, where the bulk of the magazine's subscribers lived. Of course, hardly anyone was looking at the *TV Guide* that day so I only sold 41 videos and lost thousands of dollars. Frequency equals saturation, which increases brand awareness, which increases sales.

14.   *No one* can sell a potential customer or client on your business product or service like you can – no one! *You* are your best salesperson and care far more about the success of your business than any employee ever could.

Several times in my business career I have given over key aspects of my business to an employee only to realize that the business suffered because of it. When I opened my massage school in the fall of 2000, I was running the school office while interviewing prospective teachers and handling nearly every inquiry that came in by phone and in person. I was excited about the school I was building. I knew it was going to be the best of its kind and that our graduates would be top-notch based on the curriculum and content that I had developed. When prospective students met me, they believed it too. My very first class in Olympia, Washington, was 22 students.

Around that time, I received a phone call from the owner of one of my competitors. It was a much larger school with a lot more money to spend on its new expansion campus in Vancouver, Washington. It was in an area that had a population 70% larger than Olympia. The first class that started at his new campus had only 11 students – ½ the size of mine.

The competition's new massage school location had the full power of the corporation's resources behind it, which allowed them to spend more on advertising. They also had a significant head-start with brand-awareness because they were an existing school with campuses throughout the state. Their school also had federal financial aid available to its students while I was only able to accept cash. The owner was more than perturbed. He wanted to know my secret. What was my secret? Me. That is not a boastful statement, but one based on what I *did* rather than *who* I was. This is important: I personally met with students and built a relationship with them. It made all the difference. Once again, Cory Garnaas has said countless times, "Nobody cares about your business as much as you do." Nobody. Thanks Cory!

15. You need to see yourself for who you are and realize that it is a client's privilege to do business with you. Clients will seek you out rather than you having to seek them out because you are great at what you do and you offer an exceptional, quality service to your clientele.

Do not grovel or give up your dignity so that you can keep a client. Post your policies and have new clients sign a copy of your policies along with your intake forms on their very first visit. If they do not show for an appointment or do not give enough notice to cancel, it will cost them.

When I take new clients, I ask, "How would you like to secure your reservation? I take Visa, MasterCard, Discover and American Express." If you do not have a merchant account, there are many options available to you, such as Square (see www.squareup.com). Your time is valuable and you need not be ashamed of your prices, let alone be embarrassed to charge a client a no-show fee. My only exceptions with no-show fees were related to actual sickness, or if it was the first time that the client did not show. In that case, I would remind them of my policy and let them know that I would charge if it happened again. If they called in the morning and had to cancel, on occasion, I would let them fill an afternoon slot on the same day to avoid the fee. Never be ashamed to enforce your policies.

Medical Massage Clinic Years

Everything Happens for a Reason

Immediately following my massage school training and after I had obtained my massage license in Washington State, I began to work in a salon/spa, as well as at a large health club. In a very short period of time, it became clear that most of the massage clients in the salon/spa just wanted to "feel good" and had no intention of letting me fix their aches, pains and injuries. It took me just a few months to realize that I wanted to focus all of my time at the health club.

I thoroughly enjoyed meeting and working with the client's at the club from the very first day. I had been offered the opportunity to share a massage treatment room with a woman who had been massaging at the club for a couple of decades. She was kind enough to let me massage clients and pay her a flat fee for each massage I performed, telling me the fee went to the club. The massage room that we shared was more than two decades old. It was a converted, concrete–block, storage closet. It was not great, but I loved my job and was excited about the opportunity.

Upon arrival at the club on my second day, she showed me a wound on her ankle which was about two-inches in diameter. Apparently she had taken a bad fall. I said, "You don't have *any* skin there. That white stuff you see there? That is your fascia." I knew she probably needed a skin graft, but I could not tell her that, of course, because that would be diagnosing. I *did* tell her to see her doctor immediately.

Sure enough, her ankle needed a skin graft. She underwent the procedure the following day and then spent the next month in recovery. During that month, she asked me to take care of her long-time clients. No problem. Well, there was one problem. When she returned, half of her clients decided to stay with me. She was more than upset.

As my practice grew, I found myself asking her for more and more access hours to the room, but there were not enough hours in the week. I had an idea. I asked her if she would mind if I asked the owners of the club if I could have my own room. She said, "Sure. No problem. Ask away." And I did. What she did not count on was their willingness to agree. In her mind she was certain they would refuse my offer. After all, they never offered her a new room and she had been there for 20-years before I came along.

Before I presented the owners with my proposal, I asked them if they would be open to letting me have my own room. I also asked what they were currently charging my "partner" for our shared space. I found out that they charged her less than half of what she had been charging me. Nice.

I had already surveyed the club to look for the ultimate place to make a new treatment room and found a storage closet near the glass-windowed tennis courts. It was an intersection of the tennis courts, free-weight room, adult lounge and the main hallway. It was perfect. My proposal to the club was that I would pay to tear down the storage closet, a 10ft by 14ft room, and build them an even better storage closet closer to the front, administrative offices. It would look nicer, have architectural features and wall sconces to provide better lighting for the walkway toward the indoor pool.

My office, where the old closet had been, would be new from the ground up. I even designed a soundproof wall system so that it was ultra quiet, even if kids were screaming outside the door. I would pay them a higher rate than my "partner" had paid, but apply the difference to the cost I incurred to build both rooms. When my investment was paid back, I continued to pay the new, higher rate which both the ownership and I felt was fair for a space of its kind.

It was a beautiful space. When you watch my original massage video, *Massage with Confidence*, you will see the "green room." It was complete with artistic, hand-painted faux marble, wainscoting, brass and glass light fixtures, and rich colors to match the foliage. I loved that room. My former "partner" never thought I would get my own room since I had only been at the club a short while so she was clearly unhappy. It sparked some jealousy and caused more drama than I care to write about. However, the upside was having access 7-days a week to my own room which allowed my practice even more opportunity to grow.

When I finally opened my new office, I bought a new, appointment calendar and left every space available. Sure, I would make clients believe I had to move things around in order to get them in, but I took every client at every time slot which they requested for treatment. After a few weeks, I looked at my schedule and determined when clients usually did *not* want massage. For the future, I crossed those times out as my times and days off and kept the high-demand time slots and days open for clients. Over time, I corralled my clients into the slots that were most in demand and gave myself the time off that I needed to rest and recover. In reality, I performed ten massages a day, four days a week in order to keep up with demand.

Insurance: Making a Deal with the Devil

In 1992 news began to circulate that a change was coming in how health insurance companies were going to be forced to reimburse "holistic" practitioners. The original reform came in 1993, but was reinforced and solidified in 1995 by the Washington State Legislature, requiring insurance companies to reimburse massage therapists and "other alternative" care providers who were licensed by the state's Department of Health. It was commonly referred to as the "every category" law. The day that insurance began to pay for massage therapy, the massage profession made a deal with the devil.

Although insurance reimbursements for massage is beneficial for many therapists and helps them make a livable income, the trouble is that it directly affects how the insured view massage and its inherent value. If the insured received one massage per week prior to insurance and now the policy only allows for one massage a month, trends show that they will cut back in their quantity of massage. After all, why pay insurance premiums *and* pay for massage out of pocket?

If a therapist's massage was worth $70.00 in cash prior to insurance and now it is a covered service, the value of that massage drops to the cost of the insured's co-pay. Worse yet, if your insurance company has a "preferred provider network", then you can only get massage from a pre-approved group of contracted therapists who are willing to take a drastically reduced amount for their treatment work. Just because insurance pays for it does not ensure it is the best available quality of care.

In the end, insurance coverage was not the validation massage therapists hoped we would find. Instead, it has proven to be a destructive to the value of massage as well as a restriction of access for the insured. Sad indeed.

From Health Club to Medical Office

Everything worked out well for a couple of years at the health club. That is until the owner's partnership decided that they wanted to retire and sell the club to a local business man. He was known for his cutthroat business tactics and he did not fail to live up to his reputation. Overnight, he decided that only club members could use his facility. The problem was that two-thirds of the clients that saw me for treatment were non-members, but had been referred by local physicians who themselves were members of the club. That was instantly bad for my business. Since I am not writing my memoirs, but a book about the things that have made me a better massage therapist and business owner, I will spare you the details. Suffice it to say that I moved on and began to share space with an osteopathic physician.

Early on, I realized that there was so much more to learn. He was a sports-medicine doctor who completed a sports fellowship and understood the benefits of massage more than the average doctor, even among fellow osteopaths. I made the most of every spare moment to pick his brain and learn all that I could. I was a sponge and loved the knowledge that he shared with me.

Aside from referrals from the doctor, our arrangement of sharing space proved valuable when I worked with patients who had trigger points that would not release. I would mark the trigger point with a Sharpie marker and then send the client to him for a Procaine injection (like Novocain, but designed for muscle tissue.) The trouble was it was very expensive for a physician to inject trigger points. On a lark, I made a phone call to a local acupuncturist and made him an offer. I would send him patients for acupuncture as long as he would also inject all of the trigger points that I had marked on the patient's body. It was a win-win arrangement. Clients received the same benefit from the acupuncturist and multiple injections could be performed for the price of just one injection from the doctor.

Learning from a Doctor

One of the eye-openers that I experienced while working with the osteopath is that doctors *do not* know everything. Many times he would meet with a patient and then leave the exam room to research what condition the patient most likely had. That actually made me smile. Doctors are human and we are all learning constantly. Apparently that is why they call it "practicing" medicine.

> *"Know where to find the information and how to use it - That's the secret of success" - Albert Einstein*

One final insight from my medical-office practice years and that is, not all clients want to get better or return to work! It is almost as though the injury is a rest from a job which they hate. They would rather endure physical pain than the mental and/or emotional pain of being at their job.

Bodymechanics School Years

When I set out to create the Bodymechanics School of Myotherapy & Massage, my medically-based school, I had no idea what it would entail. I spent 90-hours a week, for several months, pouring over my notes and experiences with the NCBTMB. I recalled the visits to the various schools throughout the country and tried to identify what was important vs. what was just "fluff." While I found some curriculums to be short and minimal, others were loaded with extra content and appeared to be superior to the competition. Unfortunately I also found some seemed to be based on how much the school could charge students in clinic fees and then require hundreds of hours of slave labor by those same students in order to raise revenue for the school owner!

What stunned me most was the complete disconnect between the length of a program's hours compared to the quality of its graduates. For example, if a school taught incorrect or ineffective techniques by mediocre teachers, there would be no benefit from that school's education, regardless of how many hours it offered. I have even seen graduates from Canada with over 2,000 hours of education that had no ability or confidence in performing deep tissue or injury treatment work. How can that be possible? So what is the ultimate massage curriculum length? 500-hours? 750-hours? 1,000-hours? What if those 1,000-hours were taught over only a 5-month period with no requirement for outside practice of techniques learned? Again, it is not about hours, but about what you learn and experience in your training.

One of the most important components in my program was a solid requirement for practice hours. I actually had a graduate of a 500-hour program in one of my seminars that told me she was only required to give 20-hours of massage in order to graduate. She told me that although she loved the education she received, she lacked self-confidence and palpation skills.

There were also vast differences in the philosophies and day-to-day operational ethics of schools throughout the country, which was both encouraging and discouraging at the same time. The most important question I kept asking myself was, "What does a *student* need to be exceptional upon graduation?"

That question sent me on a quest that originally seemed complicated, but was ultimately simple. If I could give my students a sound understanding of the body, help them understand how tension affects posture, what makes us move, what techniques make the most difference in the shortest time and how to truly touch a client with understanding in their hands, then I will have succeeded. Sure, I had to put the hours of each course into categories for the state vocational school license, but what the curriculum pages could not show was my passion for making the lame walk again. I love to help others and I wanted to transmit that passion into my students.

Building Confidence

Confidence for our students also came from case studies. Not studies found in a book, but from real-life case studies the student can personally be a part of and experience themselves.

During the first month that I started my school, my

girls' mother, Debbie, stopped at the horse ranch where our oldest daughter, Ashley, was volunteering. One of the other 12-year old girls, who also helped at the ranch, was scheduled to have Harrington rods installed into her spine. Debbie listened to the concerned mother's explanation of her daughter's impending scoliosis surgery and said, "Oh, Bob can fix that!"

I received a phone call from the girl's mother that evening, asking me to work my magic and "fix" her daughter's scoliosis. The truth is massage cannot "fix" scoliosis. I intended to share that disclaimer with her when I suddenly had an idea. "How old is your daughter?" I asked.

"Twelve", the mother responded.

I asked her to bring her daughter to the school and meet with me before classes the next day. When the two arrived, the mother explained that her daughter's curve was progressing and was now at 45 degrees. She was dangerously close to the "50 degree absolute progression" point and her surgeon insisted that the surgery must happen - and it had to happen *now*. I explained that although massage does not heal scoliosis, I believed we could still perform a miracle of sorts. I needed to talk with the surgeon.

The next day, I called the surgeon about the young girl's condition. I explained that I wanted to delay her surgery and start her on a treatment protocol that I had been developing. He bluntly said, "NO! She *must* have the procedure or she will certainly have life-long, dire consequences." No matter what I said, his answer was the same.

I called the mother back and told her the bad news.

She did not care. "She's *my* daughter and I want *you* to work on her. We will delay the surgery." And that was that.

The next day, the mother and daughter returned to the school. I performed a pre-assessment that was followed by a classroom demonstration and discussion for the new students in my first class.

I explained to my students, "Although we cannot change this young woman's diagnosis or remove all signs of her scoliotic curve, I do believe we can stop the condition from progressing - dead in its tracks. Although I am going to demonstrate the techniques that that she needs to have performed, I will not be providing her treatment. This is not about my skills, but about the efficacy of the technique and my theory. Even though you are brand new students and don't have much experience yet, you will be the ones who work on her, not me." I went on to explain my treatment plan, which included:

- Two, 30-60 minute treatments a week
- No soda (not only are the acids in soda hard on our bodies, the Osteoporosis Research Center reports that caffeine can leach calcium to some degree)
- She had to work with her physical therapist to get an abdominal strengthening exercise routine in place
- She had to sit up straight while at school and on the couch at night while she watched TV with her family
- She had to wear her back brace, but only to bed at night, in order to help prevent her from "sleeping funky" (aka: catawampus positioning)

After a few weeks, the mother reported that her daughter was feeling better and wanted to continue with the treatments. Two months later, she was still improving. Yet the surgeon was more than perturbed with the family's decision to disregard his orders. Our treatment protocol continued anyway.

Three months into my protocol, the young girl went back to the surgeon for "pre-surgery" x-rays. The doctor was a bit befuddled - a medical term for confusion - because upon examination the girl had a 75% *reduction* in her curvature. Did she still have scoliosis? Yes. Was she cured? No, but she never had to have the destructive surgery and only needs a monthly massage for continued, palliative care.

So why have my students do the work rather a seasoned professional? Because the students needed to see, first hand, that they were in a field that changes lives. From that point on, the Bodymechanics students had a jolt of confidence and an increased desire to learn.

Arrogance versus Overcoming Fear

I could write volumes about the thousands of massage treatments I have personally given through the years. From them I have learned about patience, humility, the effects of pride, communication challenges, ethics... the list goes on and on.

Every massage that we give contains a lesson if you look for and are open to learning and growth. During the years that I owned the school, I received many referrals asking me to treat the patients and clients that others were afraid to treat. Such as a woman I took on as a client with dual lung transplants and a broken neck. She was so happy that I made the time for her because other therapists had backed away, believing they would only make things worse. Really? When someone is in pain, I would rather "err on the side of educated arrogance" than not treat someone for fear of making things worse. If the patient wants to have your healing touch, they know their own bodies and you can do them a world of good. Should you use an elbow deeply on the spine of a 90-year old woman with advanced osteoporosis? No, of course not, however you can use common sense and give her the touch that she needs.

Due to my confidence and willingness to help others, I was also able to develop and apply my theories and observe the therapeutic results. This occurred not only with, the 12-year old scoliosis patient, but also with such diverse situations as a woman who needed help migrating her 400cc sub-pecular implant in order to make both sides match.

Careless "arrogance" *can* adversely affect your clients. I had just negotiated an exclusive program with the local AIDS network. Their clients could come to the school and receive massage free of charge. The students would volunteer their time and I would provide the linen, etc. at no cost. The program worked great until one day a new, advanced AIDS patient arrived and one of our students worked on him. The student was also an RN, but was obstinate and unwilling to listen to his instructors or to sound training. He was the nurse and I was *just* "a massage therapist"... what could I know that he did not?

The next day, I received a call from the AIDS network office. They would no longer need our volunteer students to work on their clients.

Apparently the student ignored his training, which would be to treat the patient's condition, not to display his skill set – or lack thereof. He had treated the patient like Gumby that day. He stretched him out like a healthy, athletic gymnast and ignored the patient's pleas for less pressure due to the pain he was inflicting. That poor patient could barely walk after his treatment and for several days following. I had to do some serious relationship repair because someone ignored the patient in favor of completing a technique.

All of us have training in our respective fields, but we must never lose sight of the patient. We do not necessarily do something *to* a patient, but rather, we work *with* the patient and lead them into recovery.

Accreditation

One challenging aspect of owning a vocational school was the misperceptions about "accreditation." There is a common perception that if a school is not approved for federal, student loans, it is not a good school.

At Bodymechanics we seriously considered taking our school through the accreditation process several times. Each time we began to invest in the process to become accredited by a national organization, we felt it best to back away and stop our pursuit.

Our school was accredited by the oversight board for vocational schools in Washington State by the Workforce

Training & Education Coordinating Board (WTECB). To get their approval was not easy since Washington State is one of the biggest "consumer protection" states in the nation. Schools seek national accreditation so that they can get government-backed loans for their students through the Title IV program. If we had continued to get accreditation from a national organization, such as COMTA, the process would have done two things to my school.

First and foremost, "Title IV" (government, student loans and funding program) would have required us to have the *program* approved, but not the school. Keeping our curriculum fresh and current would have been next to impossible. As a non-Title IV school, we had options and were more nimble than our competition.

Secondly, Title IV approval required that the school complete so much paperwork and additional administration hours that it would have added $2,000.00, per student, in additional tuition, just to cover our expenses. It also would have doubled my administrative staff and gave the government and credentialing bodies authority over the school in ways that were not necessarily in the student's best interest. As I told my students, there was a truck-driving school just up the road with Title IV funding. Our vocational school, located within the hospital, was a superior institution. The only way to drop the per-student expense would have been to grow by several fold, but we did not see the upside to becoming bigger.

Secrets of Success

I knew that if my students were going to succeed they needed three, specific attributes before they graduated: 1) excellent communication skills, 2) solid business and marketing training provided by a successful business person, and 3) exceptional technique based on an in-depth understanding of human anatomy, physiology and kinesiology. Even if a therapist does not have all three, it is never too late to learn and become a more successful therapist.

Destined for Working with Professionals

I loved "Creating Exceptional Massage Therapists", which was more to me than just our school's motto; it has become my personal mission. I have since realized I should have used the word "developing" rather than "creating", because it is truly up the student as to whether their excellence comes to fruition. Eventually, I also realized that school management was not for me. Students whining about missing a quiz or making excuses for not completing their practice hours drove me nuts. I wanted to work with therapists who had a thirst and desire to be exceptional, who knew that helping others through massage was their heart's passion. It became clear that teaching professional bodyworkers and health professionals through seminars was my only viable option.

Hands

Our hands are amazing tools. They can be used for good or bad, but above all else, they are only as good as their training. According to the MIT Touch Lab, each human fingertip has over 2,000 touch receptors, let alone the other receptors for pain, pressure, heat, etc. While a human hair is 50-100 microns across, your fingers have the ability to discern a 3-micron bump on a piece of glass. If I blindfolded you, gave you a Los Angeles phonebook, had you feel it, and then hid a human hair inside of that phonebook, you have the ability to actually discern the presence of that hair. Could you do that right now? Probably not. Can you learn to detect the difference? Absolutely. Touch therapists develop a greater sensitivity with experience and are better able to discern what their fingers are actually feeling below the skin.

When I was in massage school, we played a hand-sensitivity game. We took a 3ft. long piece of plastic wrap and laid it lengthwise on a massage table and then had a student sit at the end of the table while blindfolded. Another student would lay a penny, a dime, a nickel and a quarter randomly on the thin plastic wrap. The blindfolded student was told to gently "walk" their fingers on the wrap, pulling it towards them. The fingers could detect gentle tension in the plastic sheet that was created by the weight of each coin. When they thought they knew where a coin was located, they were to reach out and put their fingers on the coin without looking. The more practice the student had, the easier it was to discern the placement of each coin. The same is true with bodywork. The more you touch, the more sensory ability you have to find trigger-points, spasm, scar tissue, cysts, etc. beneath the depths of the client's skin. We literally learn to "see" with our touch.

When we opened our in-room, hospital-massage program, I was asked to be the first to go into a patient's room and run the process through its paces just as our students would. The first patient was a middle-aged man who was admitted for treatment of liver cancer. When I arrived to give him his massage, he was in his blue, hospital gown and his wife was reading the newspaper in the corner chair. "I'd like a relaxing neck and shoulder rub, if that's okay," he said.

I had him sit in a chair and began to work on his shoulders and neck. As I worked up the cervicals, I felt a 1/2" lump on the right side. I knew that cysts can often show up in the occipital and posterior areas of the neck, but I also knew what cysts feel like. This was not a cyst. I asked him cautiously, "Are you aware that you have a lump in your neck, right here?" His wife put down her paper with a concerned look. He said he was not aware. I told him not to worry himself... I was just curious.

Upon completion of his massage, I went to the nurse in charge and said, "When I was massaging the patient I noticed that he had a 1/2" lump on the right side of his neck about 2" lateral to the C-3 spinous process. You might want to have a look for yourself. I just wanted you to be aware."

My hands felt a metastasized tumor that day. What is my point? Our student, hospital-massage program was suddenly found to be more important than the hospital had realized. We could be the sensitive hands that the doctors wished they had. We do not have the knowledge of a physician, but they do not have our palpation skills. It was a great revelation for doctors in the hospital that day. As the doctors began to see the benefits with patient recovery and general well being following our student massages, they went from approving treatment on a case-by-case basis to allowing our students full access for patient massage. It was a humbling and exciting opportunity for us.

The Gift of Touch

A crucial lesson that the hospital program taught my students was that we all have an appointed time to die. If a patient's time is 11:05am tomorrow and he receives a massage from a student an hour before, it does not mean that the student killed the patient. It means that loving care from the student helped him transition into the afterlife. The student gave him a gift, not a curse. I made sure the students knew that they were agents of peace and joy, not sadness and death. We do not always know the benefits of our touch until the family sends a letter of thankfulness for the gift that you gave to their loved one. It was powerful stuff.

Theoretical Foundations of Haase Myotherapy®

Ingredients versus Recipe

Imagine a teacher walking into a classroom full of students and giving each of them an identical box of ingredients that includes sugar, flour, salt, baking soda, butter, vanilla, vegetable oils and chocolate. The teacher then asks the students to go to their respective kitchens, make something with their ingredients and then return at the end of the day to share what they made. How many would return with the very same product? Would it look or taste the same? Would it have the same consistency or moistness? No, of course not. It all comes down to the recipe - more on that later.

In massage school, you attended class with students who received the same education that you did. You all had the same school, same courses, same content, same instruction and same instructors. At the end of the training program, how many of your fellow students massaged the same way or had the same quality of technique? None. Why is that? They had the same training, but the results were different. Sure, some missed a few classes and some had dyslexia so they did things backwards, but in general, everything was the same. The *difference* is that schools, in general, teach ingredients versus a recipe.

Haase Myotherapy® is not so much about technique as it is about how to use the right technique, in the right timing and way, in order to get the optimal result. It is all about the recipe. Many of the techniques I have "made up", but I did not name them after myself. I am sure someone else accidentally stumbled upon the technique before me. For example, when I stubbed my toe last week and instinctively rubbed it because it hurt, I did not yell out, "I'm trademarking that! I claim it as the Haase Technique!"

A Lomi Lomi instructor, once said that the Hawaiians believe we are born with all knowledge, forget it at birth, and then spend the rest of our lives trying to remember it.

I asked her, "Even nuclear physics?"

"Oh yeah, even nuclear physics."

I am not sure that I entirely buy into the theory, but I will say that an intelligent massage therapist uses their knowledge of the body, combines it with their knowledge of kinesiology and movement, and then uses their hands to affect change in dysfunctional tissues. It is a natural outcome. Massage therapists "make up" techniques every day. We should not be naming them after ourselves. It makes about as much sense as saying that Christopher Columbus "found" the Americas. The locals begged to differ.

The point is, it really is not about who figured out a technique, but how that technique is used. Again, it is the recipe.

As I detailed earlier, experimenting, comparing and enhancing techniques was a huge part of my process. While in massage school, I practiced the techniques I was taught until I perfected them. Then, I would compare techniques and ask the clients two questions: 1) Which technique felt better to receive, and 2) Which technique gave them immediate and/or longer-term relief from their pain. The comparing of techniques lasted throughout my school year. One teacher was upset that I was changing the techniques which I was taught. I overheard Brian Utting, the school's owner, say in a low voice, "Leave him alone. He knows what he's doing."

Thanks for the vote of confidence, Brian.

Letting me experiment made all the difference as I continued that process into my practice. I continually compared techniques and kept the ones that worked while I tossed the less effective ones. Even with the ones that worked, I tended to tinker with and change in order to get an even more enhanced result. I also realized that there was not one type of bodywork that fixed everyone. Every condition seemed to respond differently to various types of techniques. In the end, it was clear that specific techniques were more effective than others for specific conditions.

Again, there is no single technique that cures all. You cannot apply myofascial release to the entire body and expect to get miraculous results on every body part or all soft tissue pathologies. The same goes for trigger-point release and many other types of bodywork. Remember my client and how the increase in pressure gave a different outcome? You need to find the right technique with the right recipe for the right result.

It is important to realize that my insights and perspectives on bodywork are the result of my own background, personal experiences and research. Like other instructors in our field, some come from a background in radiology, some from engineering, etc., whereas my background in autopsies gave me unique insights into deviations in human anatomy as well as the effects on human tissues as a result of injury. My experience with the Thurston County Coroner, combined with my experience in cadaver studies at Bastyr, has proved invaluable over the years and has directly impacted my theories, techniques, as well as the content and direction of the seminars I present today.

Imagine that you were asked to sit in a clear plastic chair and we positioned a camera, aiming from underneath, in order to see how gravity and pressure affected how your "butt" looked while you were in the seated position. Is it possible, even remotely, that what we would see would look slightly wider than what we would see while you were standing? Of course it would. This migration of tissue would also have a direct impact on the perspective of the artist who uses the cadaver as its artistic muse.

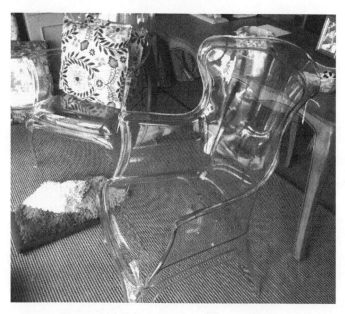

Above: The famous "clear chair" that I have been describing in my seminars for over a decade. I finally found one in Amsterdam, Holland.

Also, keep in mind that the tissues of a cadaver are extremely thin and lacking substance in relationship to the actual tissues of your clients as described earlier. Remember, anatomy books are for *general* reference. They are the same as comparing a roadmap to the open road. Keep it in perspective and trust what your hands are palpating. Sometimes the map is wrong, or at least limited by two-dimensions. .

What was interesting to me was the difference between what my expectations were compared to the realities of the body. For example, I was stunned that the brain was not as big as I had thought. When you actually cut through the scalp, into the epidermis, dermis, thick subcutaneous connective tissue, galea aponeurotica, muscles, cranial bone, dura mater, arachnoid and subarachnoid space, and then the pia mater, you finally get to the gray matter of the brain. That is a lot of thickness protecting the brain. In the end, the brain seems small compared to the entire head.

I was also stunned by how large the liver is and how much of the abdominal and lower chest cavity it consumes. It is huge, and extremely fragile compared to the other organs. But most notable was the size of the psoas muscles, as I mentioned earlier.

Years in Practice vs. Technique

Are you an honest person? Without hesitation, you would probably say "yes." The truth is, most massage therapists lie or are at least evasive when they are on a vacation and want to get a massage. The therapist gives you an intake form to fill out and you get down to the fill-in-the-blank question, "What is your occupation?" How do you answer? If you say, "massage therapist," you know you will more than likely have to discuss business during your entire massage and be unable to truly relax and enjoy. So how do you answer? Do you say, "Self employed"? I do.

Early in my career, I had made an appointment with a female therapist at a health club about 20-miles outside of my hometown. Thinking that I had dodged the "occupation" bullet, I was relaxing though my massage. That is until she unintentionally used her elbow to specifically locate each of my ribs while traveling up my back.

"Would you mind moving your elbow an inch or so medially so that you're on top of my erector spinae muscles?" I blurted without thinking.

"Are you a massage therapist?!" she excitedly questioned. "Yes." Dang it - the cat was out of the bag!

"OH! I was trained by (insert name of old-school massage therapist with very little training) and I've been a therapist for 14-years! I learned so much from her."

Moments after she told me of her training and experience, she moved to my calves. She proceeded to shove her elbow into my left gastrocnemius muscle and made a quick, deep stroke toward my foot - wrong direction! I could feel the valve in my vein collapse, which instantly left me with a varicose vein.

Did 14-years of performing an incorrect technique suddenly make it correct? No, of course not. If you were told that you needed brain surgery and had the choice between two surgeons, would you pick the surgeon who never updated the techniques he had been practicing for the past 40-years? Or would you choose a surgeon who was fresh out of a leading, medical school with state-of-the-art technique? I would choose the superior technique any day. It is not about years in practice, but about the technique and how that technique is applied to the body. It does not matter if you are 6-months or 30-years out of school. Your primary goal should be to know good technique and the best recipe for applying that technique for the maximum benefit to your client in the minimum amount of time. Are you a new therapist? It does not matter. Experienced? Again, it does not necessarily matter. What does matter is what you are doing *to* and *for* your clients.

Getting Clients Well Quickly

In Washington State, if you are injured on the job, you essentially will receive six massage treatments without much difficulty, paid for by the State's worker's compensation insurance program. If you need six additional treatments, the provider will have to write reports, contact the insurance adjuster and nearly beg. If you need six more after the first twelve, you may as well offer up your first-born child as a bribe. In other words, anything over six treatments is a huge hassle. At least it was for me. With that in mind, my goal has always been to get my clients better, out of pain and functional in six treatments or less. To make this happen, you need to work smart and have a game plan for each individual client. One treatment plan does *not* fit all.

Sadly, I have seen the "single plan" philosophy repeated in other professions throughout the country as well.

- A dentist was known for convincing every single patient that their mercury amalgam fillings must be removed in order to prevent mercury poisoning and death. Oddly, while he is replacing their original fillings with plastic, every patient coincidentally also needed at least one gold crown. And if you were wealthy, he somehow convinced you that you were in need of a platinum crown.

- An oral surgeon convinces nearly every patient (with the financial means to pay) that they are in dire need of a $20,000 oral surgery procedure, knowing full well that there are much less costly ways to treat TMJD with excellent results.

- There is a chiropractor that feels the need to take a high-quantity of x-rays with each patient, at every phase of treatment, for baseline purposes as well as to determine "effectiveness" of treatment and protocols. Since films cost very little for the chiropractor, he has tapped into a fountain of profit. Then he sells nearly every patient a set of neck and shoulder weights that cost $200.00 for the patient, but only a small fraction of that amount wholesale. He also requires x-rays of the patient with the neck/shoulder weights in place. Every one of his patients that I have spoken with has had the same protocol.

What do these three medical practitioners have in common? The same treatment was given for different clients with differing needs. It becomes routine. Sure, some patients will have miraculous results, but there are many who will not because the treatment was not truly tailored to their individual needs. If you want to get the patient better quickly, they need a treatment plan suited specifically for them.

Pain vs. Tissue vs. Psychology

One of the biggest misconceptions by "medical massage" therapists, or at least those who treat injuries, is the belief that his or her goal is simply to get the client out of pain. I disagree entirely. While the removal of pain may be what your clients are hoping for, it should not be your ultimate goal.

Imagine if a paraplegic patient comes to your office in a wheelchair and accidentally strikes their shin on the doorframe as they enter. You notice that they are bleeding from the abrasion and ask, "Are you in pain?"

"Nope."

"Okay! Then you're good to go home. Have a nice day!", you instruct as they give you a befuddled look.

The point is that we need to focus on unhealthy tissue and determine what is needed in order to treat effectively. The treatment continues until the tissues are healed, not when the patient no longer feels pain. If all we talk about is the patient's pain, that is what they are going to notice and upon which they will focus. Not only when they are in your office, but in everyday life as well.

This is even truer of fibromyalgia patients than with any other type of patient with soft tissue pain. Often, fibromyalgia patients *are* their pain. If I offered them a large nametag that said, "I Have Fibromyalgia," they would probably wear it. Fibromyalgia patients, in general, have a psychological component to their condition that makes them become one in the same with their pain, an amalgam of sorts.

They often cannot differentiate themselves from the pain. If I ask, "Hey, Janet, how are you?" The response is typically, "Oh, the pain..." They embody their pain, making it a component of their very identity.

If you took away a fibromyalgia client's pain, most would have no idea of how to act. I have a little fun with this simply to make a point with my clients. When a new fibromyalgia client comes into my office and mentions that they have the indicative "18-Points of Pain," meaning they indeed have been diagnosed with fibromyalgia, I say, "Oh dear. I, uh... I have bad news for you..."

The client looks at me with a lifted eyebrow. "What's the bad news?"

"Well, I'm going to be taking away four of your points of pain today."

The look on most fibromyalgia client's faces after I say those words is priceless. Most have a worried, almost shocked face. "What do you mean you're taking away some of my 'points of pain'?!"

I continue, "Yep. I do this for my client's all the time. You're only going to have 14-points of pain when you leave today. So... If I take away four, and you only have fourteen left... now what do you have?"

You can see it in their eyes. If you take away their label, they do not know how to behave. It is part of them. This is not a book about how to treat fibromyalgia, but I will say this: If you want to get a patient out of the endless cycle of fibromyalgia syndrome, you have to undo what they have done to themselves.

Usually, fibromyalgia patients start off with pain, so

they cannot sleep, so they do not have the energy to exercise or prepare healthy meals, so they eat poorly, starving their muscles of healthy nutrients while filling them with chemicals from "quick foods", which increases their tissue pain, so they cannot sleep... The cycle is endless. I have helped my fibromyalgia patients with a regimen that includes:

- Eating healthy, whole and raw foods, high in nutrients
- Eliminating foods that are canned, packaged or instant, and certainly not "fast food"
- Drinking one gallon of water daily
- Walking for a half-hour at a moderate pace
- Ensuring a good night's sleep.
- And lastly, get regular, as well as vigorous, lymphatic drainage work (See page 229 regarding Lymphatic Drainage). I firmly believe that most fibromyalgia patients do not eat as well as they should and end up making their tissues toxic. Even if they do eat well, removal of the toxins from the body's tissues seems to be extremely beneficial in the recovery process. Gently bouncing on a "rebounder" (mini-trampoline) for 5-minutes in the morning and 5-minutes at night really helps move the lymph. The feet never leave the rebounder; just bounce gently, at a rate of about 120 bounces a minute.

The real question is, are you only treating pain, or are you ultimately treating unhealthy tissue? Have you ever been working in the yard and had someone come up to you and say, "Oh my gosh! Your arm is bleeding."? Did you notice the abrasion before they said it? Probably not. Thanks a lot - *now* you notice it!

It is imperative that, as a therapist, you treat the conditions that cause pain, but do not focus the patient's attention on the pain. Pain is not the problem. The *cause* of the pain should be the focus.

In the movie *Up*, I loved the dog that was given a special collar that allowed it to "speak" English. The old man says, "Did that dog just say 'Hi there'?"

The dog responds, "Oh yes! My name is 'Dug.' I have just met you and I love you. My master made me this collar. He is a good and smart master and he made me this collar so that I may talk... SQUIRREL!!!" The dog's attention darts away from the old man and is now focused on nothing but the squirrel. This is distraction at its purest. Distraction helps decrease pain in many ways and especially when it comes to mental focus.

Random side note... From what I have observed, most of my patients with chronic fatigue eat extremely well and most are on self-imposed low-sodium diets. Lack of sodium reduces capillary pressure, making you feel tired. So what is the cure? Enjoy a bag of Doritos®. I like the nacho cheese flavor, but that is just me.

Also, pain tends to meander above and below a "pain threshold," of sorts. Just because you do not feel the injury, it does not mean that it is not present. This is partly due to the pain threshold and partly from the "gate theory."

Have you ever had an iron burn? It hurts like crazy. If you had a hundred iron burns on your body, simultaneously, it is unlikely that you would feel all of those burns at the same time. If I asked you, "Where does it hurt?" you might point out only a few places. But if I pushed my finger on an area that you did not point out, you would definitely notice that one as well. That explains why your clients may actually be *in more* pain upon leaving your office after their initial treatment with you. You essentially provide direct "bio feedback" and help make your client aware of what the brain had been filtering out.

Another reason why it is important to be cognizant of the fact that we are not treating pain is because our clients are usually suffering from more than one area of injury when they arrive at our offices; they just had not realized it yet. Educating your clients will help them heal more quickly as they become more aware not only physically, but emotionally and intellectually as well.

Gate Theory vs. Unwinding

Some chiropractors, myofascial release practitioners, and structural bodyworkers explain the phenomenon of pain "moving" from one location to another during a treatment series as an "unwinding" of sorts. I believe there are three common possibilities that address this phenomenon.

First is the myofascial perspective, that the body caries current and past injuries in the memory of the fascia. During a single treatment session, a client may report pain (or other sensations) in areas seemingly unrelated to where the therapist began to work. According to the MFR approach, as the body "unwinds," or releases the tension from injury due to treatment, the client becomes aware of the next area where tension is greatest in the body. The therapist then works that area of the body based on client feedback and/or visual confirmation of change in fascial/muscular tension throughout the body. Treatment progresses in that manner throughout the session. The theory is that there can be a continuous unwinding, bringing the body into tensional balance and structural relaxation. I address MFR approach this more in depth later in this book on page 235.

The second possibility is that of muscular stabilization as a result of compensation, which can cause pain to seemingly "move" throughout the body with ongoing treatments. For example, if a patient stubs their toe, they may limp, which forces other structures out of balance and causes an adaptive response. As the therapist works to release compensating muscular tension, the muscles that had to adapt and compensate the most no longer have to take on the additional workload or adjust for variations in muscles tension. As this restoration of movement and balance of workload is achieved, the compensating muscles will likely require treatment to alleviate fatigue and pain. This is also an "unwinding", usually noticed by the client over time.

However, more often than not, patients are dealing with a situation of "what hurts most." That is, a revelation of sorts, revealing that which had been previously blocking awareness of other underlying injuries. For example, once you assist the neck recover, then the hip begins to hurt. So you treat the hip and as it gets better, the shoulder starts to hurt. Did the shoulder have issues all along, as well as the neck and hip? More than likely, but the patient was not aware of the pain because the neck hurt more than the other areas and the "gate theory," a protection mechanism, blocked the client from feeling the associated pain.

Do you ever wonder why a patient arrives with a prescription in hand that says, "Treat 6X for Cervical Sprain and Strain"? Usually it is because that patient went to their doctor after an accident and said, "My neck hurts." The problem is, when the patient presents to you with that prescription, you will be tempted to work everything that hurts. I strongly suggest that the therapist should *not* treat any other area than what is prescribed, if they are billing an insurance company. When you work outside the confines of that prescription, it becomes problematic when you write chart notes and bill the insurance companies. Red flags go up when the adjuster reads that you did not follow the prescription and they may deny payment on the claim. My suggestion is to treat the neck, as requested, but palpate all the other areas as well. Then write the referring physician a report with your findings along with your treatment plan recommendation.

It might read something like this:

Dear Dr. Smith,

Thank you for your referral of Mike Doe for treatment of his cervical injuries sustained during his motor vehicle accident (MVA) on January 15, 2011. Per your request, I have treated Mr. Doe's cervical areas and indeed found the right, posterior cervical group to be in exquisite tenderness upon palpation. Cross-fiber treatment, along with trigger point therapy and muscle energy techniques, followed by ice, seemed not only to provide him some relief, but also increased cervical range of motion.

In addition to the treatment provided, I palpated other muscular and soft tissue areas that are likely involved as a result of injury during Mr. Doe's MVA. I have noted the following upon palpation:

Key:

B = Bilateral

L = Left

R = Right

SP = Spasm

TP = Trigger Point

= Pain level on a 1-10 scale, with 10 being the worst pain possible

- *Trapezius, B-R-SP-7*
- *Pectoralis Minor, B-R-TP & SP- 7*
- *Psoas, B-L-8-SP*
- *Quadratus Lumborum, B-R-8-SP*

- *Posterior Cervical Group, B-L-SP & TP*
- *Deep Anterior Cervicals (Omohyoid, Thyrohyoid), B-TP-6*

With your approval, I would like to treat all of Mr. Doe's soft tissue injuries simultaneously, thereby reducing his overall treatment regimen, cost to the insurance company and missed time and wages from work. In addition to the cervical sprain and strain treatment, I would recommend treating the above-noted muscles twice a week for two weeks, once a week for three weeks, once every ten days for thirty days and a follow-up treatment two weeks later. This would be eleven additional treatments, for a total of twelve treatments in the protocol.

If you concur, please confirm with your signature below and return the top copy for our records.

   Sincerely,

   Robert B. Haase, LMP
   ☐ *Treatment Plan Approved as requested*
   ☐ *Please treat per original Rx*
   ☐ *Please treat per this revised plan:* _____

   _____

   _____

   Physician Signature: _____

The great news is that doctors love massage therapists because we can be their hands. Doctors are required to know a lot of information, but muscular palpation and the ability to determine which muscle they are feeling is not within most of their skill sets. If you can provide them with a report after seeing their patient and identifying your specific palpatory findings, they will gladly receive your input.

I still chuckle when I recall the time I was massaging a doctor who had graduated from a top-notch, medical school in the USA. As I worked on his psoas, I said, "Wow, Doc. Your psoas muscle is really tight."

"No, Bob, that's the 'illiopsoas' muscle."

"No, Doc, it's just the psoas."

"No, Bob, it's actually the 'illiopsoas."

"Actually, Doc, your illiacus and your psoas muscles are both agonists and flexors of the hip. Both muscles spin into each other and connect at the same point on the lesser trochanter of your femur, but just your psoas is tight today..."

"Oh."

The good doctor realized that although he memorized muscle names and had a pretty good idea of where most of them were, he really did not *know* the muscles. Just like the pathologist at the coroner's office, muscle awareness falls into the massage therapist's purview, but not typically a medical doctor's.

I have already mentioned the "pain threshold." It is important that your clients understand what the pain threshold means to them. On the client's first visit, I always explain, as I draw on a piece of paper, that there is this invisible line that is unique for each person when it comes to feeling pain. When there is injury or some type of tissue problem that intensifies the pain, it rises above that line and the person actually feels pain. When the issues resolve somewhat or the brain is distracted, the client does not feel it. Typically, when they no longer feel the pain, they stop treatment and cease to recover properly.

Again, it is imperative that every new client realizes that we are not in the business of treating pain, but injured tissue. If a client discontinues treatment before the tissues are fully healed, the injured tissues can exacerbate from simple, everyday activities. A month later, the client will be back on your doorstep, angry because they are dealing with the same "stuff" and *you* must not have done your job correctly in the first place or else the pain would not have returned! Of course this is faulty logic on the client's part, but if you educate them upfront, you will undoubtedly have a much more compliant client.

Symptom vs. Source

From where does pain come? Have you ever heard the expression, "No brain, no pain"? It is true. Pain is felt in the brain and it is a symptom of unhealthy tissue. My hope is that you use pain as an *indicator* that something is wrong. The truth is that most people point to the symptom, not the problem.

This might sound a bit absurd, but it provides a perfect example. If a patient walked in the door while unknowingly having a heart attack and told his massage therapist that his chest hurt and he had pain going down his arm, the massage therapist might say, "Let's massage your chest and arm! That'll fix it!"

The chest and arm pain are the *symptom*, not the problem.

If a client walks into a massage office with their shoulders rounded forward and indicates that they have a headache at the base of their skull, a bad massage therapist probably says, "I'm going to massage your big toe!" A good therapist says, "I hear you. I'm going to massage what hurts!" And they proceed to massage the neck and head. However, a great therapist asks the client about contributing factors that have lead to his dysfunctional posture, which is causing the pain. They would also ask specific questions about the pain. Such as, is the pain constant throughout the day or only at certain times? Do certain activities exacerbate the headache? Great therapists ask questions in order to develop a treatment plan before initiating treatment because there is almost always more to the story than just pain.

In reality, people seldom feel pain at the site of the problem unless there is a direct injury to those tissues. Just as in a bad relationship, the bully in the relationship seldom feels any pain. The abused partner usually does.

In bodywork, less knowledgeable therapists often focus on and treat only the abused and leave the abuser alone, which allows the perpetuation of abuse. This strategy is great for business, but bad for the client. We need to determine the cause of the pain, educate the client as to why you are treating the opposite area of where they feel the pain, and then restore the muscles to a healthy, balanced relationship by utilizing the appropriate recipe for   treatment.

Tensegrity and Posture

People are very much like circus tents.   Of course they do not like to hear that, so I tell them that they are a very "thin and svelte" circus tent, but a tent nonetheless. The term is called "tensegrity," or tensional integrity. When your client understands this concept, they are much more likely to understand why you are working deep in their abdomen when they have presented for treatment of lower back pain. I tell them, "Like a circus tent, the body has poles, ropes and tarp. The poles are your bones, the ropes your muscles and the tarp your skin and fascial network. If the ropes are tighter on one side of the tent, the tent leans toward that direction. However, if the ropes are overly tight on all sides, the tent stands upright, but the poles are getting damaged."

This principle is very important when it comes to understanding the symbiotic relationship between massage and chiropractic. You cannot have a circus tent that uses poles without ropes, nor can you use ropes by themselves without a pole to create the lift. The same is true for the human body.

If you were only made up of muscles, you could flex them all for a few seconds in order to stand up, but you would quickly tire and fall to the ground. If you were simply bones without muscles, you would tip over like "pickup sticks."

When a person says that they believe in massage but not chiropractic, they are just as mistaken in their thinking as a person who believes in chiropractic and not massage. Sure, you can force a joint into submission that is suffering from a fixation, but if it is under extreme pressure from muscle tension, you will risk damaging that joint.

In the case of the circus tent, if you want to move a pole, you must first loosen the ropes. By the same reasoning, massage should always precede the adjustment. From my experience, there is a marked decrease in the overall number of treatments if the massage is performed just prior to the chiropractic adjustment. This is because relaxed muscles are less likely to guard - which would force the fixation to immediately return.

As a side note, I disagree with the term "subluxation" as it has been used by chiropractors throughout the past century. According to the Association of Chiropractic Colleges (ACC), "subluxation" is defined as:

"Chiropractic is concerned with the preservation and restoration of health, and focuses particular attention on the subluxation. A subluxation is a complex of functional and/or structural and/or pathological articular changes that compromise neural integrity and may influence organ system function and general health. A subluxation is evaluated, diagnosed, and managed through the use of chiropractic procedures based on the best available rational and empirical evidence."

In reality, the issue is more of a "fixation" when a client is dealing with a spine that is considered "out of alignment." The "fixation" is when two vertebrae are not moving as well as they should. This is also true with the joints and muscles. When two vertebrae are fixated and not moving correctly, the local metabolism of a joint is affected, creating a toxic environment, which in turn is caustic to the associated nerve. Often, the pain felt is from that caustic effect on the nerve roots rather than because the joint in "subluxation. "

According to the medical profession, a true subluxation is a partial or complete dislocation of a joint or organ. If a person truly had subluxation of their spine, they would likely be paralyzed.

If you ask ten chiropractors to explain their opinion on this, you will likely get ten different responses. In reality, there is no clear agreement in the chiropractic profession and this topic has been known to be explosive amongst chiropractors in general.

As I have long said:

> *Movement is Life... Lack of*
> *Movement is Death.*

In school, you may have learned how to measure a client's postural deviations with a grid-type, wall chart or a plumb-bob. Have you ever noticed how you adjust your car's rear view mirror in the morning and then often need to readjust it at the end of the day? Did you shrink? No, but your posture changed due to fatigue.

We would all agree that a raised shoulder is an obvious sign of muscle tension. Consider then, if every muscle in your body were simultaneously in spasm, in theory, you would have perfect posture. Did you read that twice? Spasms can lead to perfect posture! With that in mind, how important are postural measurements? What if you were to measure a client this morning and then again tomorrow afternoon? They may appear to be getting worse. Reverse that order and you may get a false sense of satisfaction from change that may have never truly occurred. I tell my female clients not to buy shoes in the morning because they will be tight by the afternoon or evening. Always buy shoes at the end of your day if you want them to have the wiggle room needed due to potential swelling.

My point is this: Do not put too much stock into measuring your client's posture. Instead, use postural observations as general insights into obvious imbalances. Notation that a client has a "2% improvement in posture" is ridiculous because our posture changes that much during the course of a day from fatigue alone.

Please take a moment and do me a favor - an experiment of sorts. Do NOT move... seriously! Hold still! Now, pay attention to your neck as you are reading this book. How does it feel? Lock that sensation into your memory. Now, I want you to sit up straight and tilt your head backward as far as you are able. Look up and let the effect of gravity take hold while the weight of your head drops your head down. The longer you hold this position, the more you will feel the heaviness of your head. You will begin to feel increased tension along with some discomfort. You will more than likely feel the effects of old injuries creeping back. Hold this position for about 30-seconds.

Now, slowly let your head fall forward as you bring your chin to your chest. Do you feel the increase effect of gravity? Do you feel the weight begin to intensify? The longer you hold this position, the more you will again feel the aches and pains return due to old injuries to your neck. Hold this position for about 30-seconds, and then return your head to a neutral, upright position.

As you bring your head up, stop at just the point where you do not feel inclined to fall forward or backward. As you find that neutral spot, your head should feel nearly weightless. Now, is your head in the exact same position as it was before you started this experiment? Most likely it is not. That means you have been using your muscles as anchors rather than movers - essentially you have been causing yourself unnecessary pain and discomfort. If *you* are holding your head this way, considering that you are an aware and educated healthcare practitioner, how much more likely is it that your clients and patients are as well? Neck stress and pain are often related to posture more than any other cause.

This will be discussed more at length under the section called **Perpetuating Factors**, but it is important to note that many clients place themselves in horrific postural situations, which not only cause, but also exacerbate their pain. I had a client with significant anterior flexion and subsequent headaches. When I asked her about her sleep habits, she bragged that she "spoils" herself with three pillows at night. Yes, she said *three!* She refused to listen to the obvious fact that 8-hours of anterior flexion while sleeping has been causing her distress. Clients are often their own worst enemy.

Show Me Your Pain

There are three types of soft tissue pain, which we commonly encounter as massage therapists. Most can be detected by how the client demonstrates their pain as they point it out on their own body. While it is important to have a client identify their pain on an intake form by marking it on a representative figure, it is just as important to have them also show you the pain on their body by pointing to it. *How* they show you is very telling.

- If the client points, with their finger, to their pectoralis major and says, "It hurts right there", there is probably an injury to the tissues at that very spot.
- If the client holds the muscle while pressing on it and says, "It hurts here", they are more than likely dealing with an antagonistic muscle fight and are pointing to the abused muscle.
- If the client uses their hand to "paint" on the pain by rubbing or brushing an area, more than likely they are dealing with a referred- pain pattern from trigger points.

Again, *how* they demonstrate their pain is the key and can provide you with insights about how to proceed with your massage treatment. It is also interesting to note the pen pressure used while the patient marks the painful areas on their intake form. If they press the pen deeply into the paper and almost tear the paper as they circle their pain, there is more than likely a psychological component to their pain. They may even become angry while discussing their pain.

The good news is that once the pain is gone and the

tissues have healed so that they are able to function normally again, their demeanor will usually return to what it was prior to the injury. If someone enters your office in a bad mood, realize that it probably has nothing to do you. On some occasions, a client's personality has shifted so severely due to the prolonged, intense pain   that I have had to refer them to a counselor in order to help them cope with the "inconvenience" of their pain and how it has affected their quality of life.

The Importance of Your Words

It is essential that you realize how important your words are as well as the power that those words hold. Recall the earlier exercise when I had you tilt your head back, then forward and mentioned you may feel the effect of old injuries? When I do this exercise in my seminars, I am cautious not to put too much emphasis on what the student is likely feeling. I came to realize that I was actually giving attendees headaches through the power of suggestion. My word choices, including the way in which I described what they might be feeling, were in a low, gentle voice, which is considered hypnotic. I should have known better.

You see, my father was a lieutenant in the US Navy while I was a young boy. As a supply officer, he would go out to sea on deployment for six-months at a time, and had to leave my mom and us kids behind. This was in the days before Skype, email and Tivo. So Dad did not have much to do except "conversate" with his fellow crew members and read books. Although Dad began his interest in hypnosis while he was a college student, he perfected his skills with continued study while at sea.

In short, my father read book after book about hypnosis and the amazing power of suggestion. He practiced the techniques on fellow students and later fellow officers. Ultimately he became exceptional with hypnotic suggestion. As a matter of fact, he became so good that he was asked to entertain Navy personnel while at sea. The stories of Dad's performances have reached the stuff of legends. The point is, my father taught me at an early age about the power of

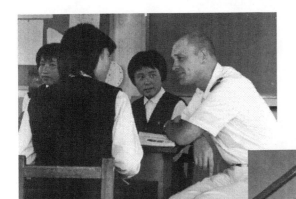

Above: My father, Lieutenant Robert Leo Haase, teaching Japanese students English while on tour in Japan in 1965.

Right: Mom and Dad while stationed in Hawaii, 1965.

Below: Me and my father on Father's Day, 2009.

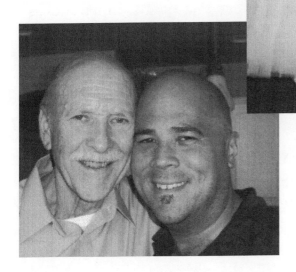

suggestion and the power of my words. I am not talking about quantum physics and the power of my thought, but actual suggestion to the human brain.

For example, I would be willing to wager a bet that there is someone's name that I could mention to you that would give you a spontaneous headache, or feeling of stress or aggravation, as soon as the name left my lips. It could be an ex-spouse, business partner, or political figure, just to name a few.

My point is, if my words can *cause* you pain, my words *can also* alleviate pain. Understand that your words can affect your clients, both for good and bad. Specifically, words most directly affect the muscles. They may also affect bone, but only nominally by comparison.

Muscles are directed by the brain - the very same brain that thinks and *listens*. When my brain tells my body to relax, the body does not have much option other than to obey. How your clients perceive the work that you do with them during their massage treatment is directly affected by your words as well as by the therapy itself. If a client presents with lower back pain and you intend to use the Haase Myotherapy® lower back release with them, you have several choices of how you present your intentions.

- You can say in a dejected voice, "Well, I learned this new lower-back technique, but it probably won't work." That is a negative tone, which gives the client little hope of improvement.
- Or you can state in a neutral voice, "I learned this new technique for lower back pain. Let's give it a try." – This

will give the client a neutral shot at recovery.

- *Or,* you can excitedly proclaim, "OH! I'm so excited! I learned this amazing technique where nearly everyone gets better within minutes! It's awesome and I'm so excited for you! Come on... let's get you out of pain! As a matter of fact, I am so sure you're going to feel better that I won't charge you if you don't feel better!" Now *that* is a powerful example of positive speech and the most likely way for your technique to have maximum benefit for your client.

Consider also that words affect emotions. When a person hears speech that is hurtful or negative, the resulting strong emotions can affect the person's physical posture in an adverse way. When people are "beat down" with negative words they often take on a fetal or cowering posture. That negative posture puts stress on the body which can cause the client pain and other adverse symptoms.

People also cower into a defensive (i.e. fetal) position when feeling threatened or unsafe. That position either comes from, or causes, the sympathetic nervous system to click-on the "fight or flight" mode. If the sympathetic engages because of negative speech, the result may be a cowering posture. Even the *position* of cowering can lead to the sympathetic response through instinct. In other words, either can initiate the other. Cowering posture does not only occur while standing. It can also be present while sleeping in the fetal position or sitting at a desk with slumped shoulders. The position itself can elicit the fight or flight mode.

The danger to the person who has a prolonged engagement of their sympathetic nervous system is the resulting altered brain chemistry due to the negative chemical cascade that results. The prolonged exposure of the brain to the negative chemicals will ultimately require intervention in order to restore balance and health. While the preferable answer is bodywork, nutrition and counseling, some cases might temporarily require medication to compensate for the altered mental state. Be sure to have a list of providers available for proper referral.

While we can help a client dealing with direct adverse affects from negative speech, we need to realize that in order for them to realize full recovery, the negative speech needs to be addressed. Let your words be the first tool in your tool belt to help *you* get your clients on the road to recovery. Your words can affect a client's *beliefs*, which affect their treatment outcome, which leads into our next topic... The powerful affects of placebo.

The Power of Placebo

When a pharmaceutical company wants to get a new drug approved, they have to run a drug study, or "human trials." Part of that study includes a "control" group, which gets no medication whatsoever. The other two groups are the "placebo" group and then the group that receives the actual medication. The placebo group is treated the same as those that receive the real drug, but they do not know it and neither does the physician. This is what is known as a "double-blind study." However, simply by the patient believing that they may be receiving the real drug gives them some level of benefit. This is called the "placebo effect" which proves the incredible power of our thoughts.

Over the years, medical study after medical study has proven that placebos are often nearly as powerful as the actual drug that is being tested for efficacy. Again, just the *thought* that one is receiving a new, ground-breaking drug has the brain producing positive results. Faith, hope and expectation are powerful drugs, but you will not find them on your insurance company's approved formulary.

Studies using "placebo surgeries" have produced positive results as well. These studies utilized a control group, a placebo group that received a "sham" surgery and the group that received the actual surgical procedure. Those with the placebo surgery are actually cut open and then sewn shut, which makes the patient believe that he had the real deal. It also allows for any potential benefit from anesthesia, or the like, to be removed from the equation. The only problem with the placebo surgeries is that sometimes they work too well! In numerous studies, placebo surgeries have proven to be just as effective, if not more effective, than the real surgery. Why? Again, it is the magic of faith, hope and expectation. As a therapist, your excitement has a direct affect on your client's expected outcome and rate of healing. If you have an ethical problem with that, then simply offer a money-back guarantee. If your treatment does not work, do not charge the client.

Your words before, during, and after a treatment should be focused on the positive outcome your patient will experience. You may have been told it is best to be quiet while massaging someone. That is good advice if you are in a spa environment. However, if you are treating a client's injuries in a clinical environment where you are free to communicate - speaking positively is *crucial*.

It is also important to give realistic expectations about when the client will feel the benefit. For example, just because you stop banging your "funny bone," it does not mean that the pain stops immediately. It usually takes one to two days to feel the full effect from nerve impingement release. However, my lower back treatment is instantaneous and the client feels relief the moment that they climb off of the massage table! I am clear with all of my clients about when they will feel better and/or how long they may feel discomfort from the treatment itself. "You're going to cuss my name tomorrow, but you're going to love me in two days!"

When my words come true, they respect me, but they respect the therapy that I provide even more. When the pain is gone, as promised, they are eager to tell a friend.

Here is an example of how positive speech can be put into practice. Over the years, I have given *free* carpal tunnel treatment to hundreds of people. It has been a great business builder, but has also made me a few enemies within the surgical community.

Whenever I am at the grocery store and see a cashier wearing a carpal or wrist brace, I always ask this question:

"Carpal tunnel?"

"Yeah. It isn't any fun."

"Are you scheduled for surgery?"

"I am, in about two weeks."

"Look, I'll make you a deal. I'm an injury–treatment massage therapist. I will give you two 5-minute treatments in a 7-day period and won't charge you a dime. If it doesn't make all of your symptoms go away, I'll give you fifty bucks."

Their mouth usually drops open at this point. Then they ask for clarification, "Let me get this straight. You want to give me two treatments. Free. No charge. And, if I'm not completely better, *you're* going to pay *me* fifty dollars??"

"Yep. That's my offer. Here's my card."

"Look, I'm confused. Why would you do that?"

"Oh, that's easy. You see, I've been doing this a long time and all but two of my clients over the years have cancelled their surgeries because I gave them just two 5-minute treatments. When you get better from my doing this simple fix, a number of things are going to happen:

1. You are going to get complete relief within the next 7-days
2. You will call to cancel your surgery and tell your surgeon that you are pain free (asymptomatic)
3. Your surgeon is going to be upset with me because he's missing another one of his boat payments because you no longer need his surgery
4. You will tell your friends what happened and they will ask for my number, wanting me to treat what ails them"

"It's a win-win. You're pain free without a destructive surgery and I build my business. You've got my card, call me as soon as you're off of work today."

I tell clients what to expect and then deliver. Too many therapists perform a massage treatment and say, "cool" when the client says that they are pain free as a result of treatment. It is almost as if the massage therapist is surprised that their massage made a difference. If the therapist is surprised and the client is surprised, then you both have lost. You will have diminished the value of your services and may have cost your client greater potential recovery because of your words and lack of faith in your abilities.

Utilizing this principle has literally been a lifesaver outside of the office environment as well. Words are important not only for the benefit of others, but for you as well. For those who know me, they know I am not a crystal-carrying, energy-embracing therapist. So what I am about to say may seem odd to them.

Working for yourself typically does not include the benefit of "sick-leave", so days off hurt the pocketbook much more than for those who work for larger companies. When I first became a therapist, I seemed to pick up every flu, cold, pain and emotion from which my clients suffered. This was not good for business, or my health, until I remembered the power of the brain over the body. Let me take you back a few years with three stories that will explain this idea a little better.

37-years ago: I was spending the night at a friend's house and his mother gave me a feather pillow. I was about 12-years old, at the time. Prior to that day, feather pillows caused my eyes to glue shut, overnight, from an allergic reaction. That night, however, I decided that I was not going to be allergic to down feathers any longer. "Thank you," I smiled as I took hold of the pillow. I love feather pillows." Were my eyes covered in glue the next day? Nope. Not a trace of glue. I was fine.

12-years ago: My family took a weekend road trip to the coast of Washington State. We stopped at a remote resort for lunch. The family was busy with multiple conversations (just like any other meal) while my youngest daughter, Holly, was eating the potato chips which came with her children's meal. Her older sister, Ashley, started reading the package ingredients out loud, "potatoes, peanut oil..." Everyone at the table froze. Five-year old Holly was deathly allergic to *anything* with peanuts in it, including peanut oil. My baby looked at me with a knowing face. Everyone else had stopped breathing. I looked at Holly and said, "Holly, you are not going to have a reaction to these chips. This is a special kind of peanut oil and you can't get sick from them. You will be fine. Do they taste good?" Miles from the nearest medic or hospital, Holly enjoyed her lunch without an anaphylactic reaction!

9-Years ago: My buddies and I were in New York City at an amazing Chinese restaurant located in an upscale part of Lower Manhattan. It is always a good sign when 80% of the customers are Chinese and wearing nice suits. It was the kind of place where you each ordered what you wanted and the waiter would serve a little of each entree onto each person's plate, then cleared away the serving bowls. After we each ordered something, I left to go to the restroom to wash my hands. I did not realize that my friends had ordered one more entree in my absence. When the meal arrived and we were all served, I took a big bite of this large, round, white thing on my plate. It was amazing! I gulped it down and said, "Wow! What is that?" My friend responded, "That's a giant scallop." I paused and then smiled as I said, "Normally I would go into anaphylactic shock from eating this, but I'm going to be fine. This tastes amazing." My friends looked at me with raised eyebrows. Sure enough, no reaction.

What do these three stories have in common? They all go back to my father's hypnotism days. As a young boy, he had told me that he could actually convince people, while under hypnosis, that a hot iron had just burned them. The skin would actually raise and look red due to a local, histamine reaction!

Our thoughts *do* control the physical body more than we realize. I applied this concept to my work. I realized that if I could just visualize myself working on my clients through the rubber gloves of an invisible incubator, then I would not get sick or pick up on their emotional energy. It worked. From the first day that I believed that, I have never gotten sick from my clients or picked up on their emotional pain again. Your words affect your own body as well as the bodies of others.

Please use common sense with this information. I am not suggesting you put your life or the lives of others at risk by not seeking appropriate medical attention or by purposely putting yourself in harms way.

Theory: Less Touch = Faster Response

The less a muscle is touched, the faster it responds to touch.

Read that again...

The *less* a muscle is touched, the *faster* it responds to touch.

Your hand, by design, is touched daily. Hand massage feels good, but it usually does not yield significant discernible change in the tissues as a client experiences hand massage.

However, when you work the psoas, located deep within the abdomen, you will get a prompt response because it is seldom touched. The same is true when we work the longus colli and longus capitis, located deep inside the neck, beneath the trachea. This follows the logic of desensitization.

We can utilize the desensitization principle while we work with a client who is exquisitely tender to even the slightest touch. When I have a client who is overly sensitive, I simply brush my hand quickly over their skin, back and forth, as though I am brushing off some dust. As I continue this quick, brushing stroke, the area becomes desensitized and allows me to work with increased pressure yet less perceived discomfort. But remember, now that you have desensitized the tissues, it will take more work in order to achieve a response.

Have you ever had a client who was comfortably lying on your massage table, but when you began to put the slightest pressure on their skin they lurched in pain? "OH MY GOD! That's too much pressure!" they will scream. Usually, it is the fibromyalgia patient. I may be only applying two ounces of pressure, yet they scream out in pain. As mentioned previously, there is a psychological aspect to fibromyalgia and seemingly a mental disconnect as well. The brain is receiving misinformation. I will ask the patient, "How did you get here today?"

"I drove."

"Did you hover over your car seat as you drove here?"

"No."

"Were you screaming out the window at the top of your lungs as you drove here?"

"No. Why are you asking me that?

"Well, I am only applying this much pressure (I push gently on her forearm with the same pressure as I applied to her back) and you are saying it is unbearable. The truth is, there was more pressure on your backside while you were driving here than what I am applying now. Your nerves are lying to your brain. I need to help reset your perception of reality."

At that point, I begin to brush the skin, in order to desensitize it, which allows me to do my work and help the client's health improve.

Let us hold to the "the less a muscle is touched..." thought for a moment as I add an additional thought to the mix...

Warm Up Theory

In school, you were likely told to "warm up the tissues before going deep." This theory is great, unless you are working on an acute injury that is already "warmer" than it should be due to inflammation. Tissues that are in the acute phase of injury are typically inflamed. Imagine if your client had a sunburn on top of a muscle that was in spasm. Would you work the muscle for a while, first, to warm it up prior to going in deep? Or would you think, "Maybe I ought to just work the problem and be done with it." The truth is that the tissues are already inflamed and, as I explain in the discussion about hydrotherapy (see page 225), it is important to *arrest* the inflammation versus feed it.

Now, let us put those two thoughts together... 1) The less a muscle (tissue) is touched, the faster it responds to touch and 2) Do not "warm up" an area that is already inflamed in the acute stage. What am I suggesting? When you are dealing with an acute injury, do not warm up the area. Instead, sink in, perform the treatment, get out and then *ice* the area in order to arrest the inflammation. That is it. If you warm it up first, you add fuel to the fire, increasing present inflammation while desensitizing the tissues at the same time. In the end, warming up already inflamed tissues results in the necessity for additional treatment.

Psychological Desensitization

Two additional thoughts are needed about "desensitization." Not desensitization of the tissues, but a desensitization of the brain.

In my early years of practice I worked on a woman who had been sexually molested from the ages of 5 until 9-years. She had been brave enough to tell her mother that her mother's boyfriend was touching her in a "bad way." Even though her mother did not believe her, somehow the touching stopped.

Twenty-years after she experienced the abuse, she was on my table requesting deep tissue massage. While I worked on her back, it did not seem to matter how deeply I worked, she wanted more pressure. As I started to press my reinforced thumbs into her infraspinatus muscle, she said, "You can go deeper." So I did. "You can go deeper," she said again. I pushed with more pressure on that muscle than I had on any previous client. She asked for me to go deeper yet. And I did. That is when I heard it.

If you were a child in the 1960's through 1970's, you may remember playing with a particular toy made of metal. I called them "clickers." You would depress the metal until it made a clicking sound. As I pushed deeper, the flat part of her shoulder blade, the infraspinous fossa, clicked. The web of bone on this healthy, 29-year old woman's scapulae literally snapped down and back up, just like the metal clicker of my childhood.

She again asked for me to go deeper. I had to tell her that I could not go any deeper without damaging her tissue. That day, in my 2nd year as a massage therapist, I realized the power of sexual and emotional abuse on the human body. Unfortunately, she was the first of many clients over the years who have demonstrated a desensitized perception of their own bodies - a detachment of sorts. When abuse occurs, (whether physical, mental, emotional or a combination of these traumas), we humans have a self-defense mechanism that kicks into gear and guards us from feeling any further pain.

A few years ago, while teaching at a seminar in Texas, a tall, Amazon-like woman volunteered to be the demonstration model for my deep adductor technique. As I worked on her, I isolated one of the tightest adductor magnus muscles that I had ever encountered on a client. As I worked deeply, I commented, "This must really be uncomfortable."

"No, I don't feel anything."

I thought she was joking. Anybody with that much tension would be in tears from the pressure. "Are you serious? You don't feel anything?"

"Nope."

I chuckled and jokingly said, "Going through a divorce are you?"

"I am divorced."

Normally, I would follow with a tableside discussion of how emotional, physical or sexual trauma can desensitize us to how we perceive touch, especially during a massage. Something deep inside me said to bite my tongue and forego that discussion.

A week later, she sent me an email and shared with me that she had not been completely honest with me. She recounted a difficult story about how she had experienced two separate incidents of rape in the years prior to meeting me at the seminar. As a result of the traumas, she lost sensation in parts of her legs, including her inner thighs, and was currently unable to run due to instability of the pelvic region. She knew that the rapes had caused not only physical injury, but emotional and spiritual injuries as well.

I was able to connect her with a gifted, male, massage therapist who generously offered to work with her without pay. Together they were able to address her emotional, physical, and spiritual traumas and achieve complete healing. Today she is able to run again and fully enjoy life, which includes experiencing the joys of intimate touch. Is that not awesome?! I love it when people are restored through caring and nurturing touch.

Injuries and Interviews

Years ago, a 17-year old girl walked into my office for a deep tissue treatment. The conversation began simply enough. "I hear you're good with fixing people's backs. Can you fix mine?"

She appeared healthy and wore a big smile. Although she was obviously uncomfortable and seemed a little apprehensive that the rumors about how I could help get her get out of pain could actually be true. Her expectations had been dashed before.

I asked her, "How long have you had back pain?"

"Three years."

"Wow. Since you were fourteen years old? You've had back pain since you were fourteen?"

"Yes."

The look in her eyes told me everything - she had lost hope. "What have you tried over the past three years to get out of pain?"

Her response was not what I had expected. "Well, the list of what I haven't tried is shorter, but..." She took a deep breath and said, "I've been treated by a medical doctor, naturopath, two chiropractors, a physical therapist, massage therapist, acupuncturist, and a surgeon."

"A surgeon?"

"Yep. He took out my tailbone. It's in a jar at home. You want to see it?"

"No, I'm good. No need."

I was frustrated for her. If all of these intelligent people had worked on her and they still could not figure it out, the answer must be something simple. Sometimes the hyper-intelligent overlook the obvious. I knew I was going to have to dig and ask the right questions in order to uncover what no one else had up until that point. The onset of the pain had to lie somewhere in her "perpetuating factors."

I asked her, "What did you do three years ago that you can't do now?"

Her eyes got big and lit up. "Horses! I *love* horses! I used to ride all the time and even competed, but I can't now."

I did not know much about horses, but I asked.

"Did you 'gallop'?"

"We call it 'cantering,'" she stated matter-of-factly.

"Oh." I stood corrected. All I could visualize was her on her horse, posting (holding herself nearly weightless in her saddle). I could see her knees bent, hips flexed, and the stress of the muscles as she made the observer believe it was effortless.

It had to be her psoas muscle. "Has anyone ever worked on your back pain through your stomach?"

"Why would they do that?" she asked.

"Just curious. Lay face-down on my massage table."

I began by releasing the abused quadratus lumborum muscle and then had her carefully turn over so that I could work her psoas. I worked with intensity, yet within her pain threshold. After no more than five minutes of treatment, I helped her carefully sit up and then get off of the massage table. As soon as her feet hit the ground, she began to cry. I get that a lot. I must have said, "Crap," out loud, because she immediately said, "NO! No, I'm okay. I'm crying because I'm happy... the pain is gone!"

I tried to maintain my smile, but honestly, I was angry

that so many healthcare professionals had taken her family's money, her precious time, and literally years from her life due to unnecessary and prolonged pain. No one had asked her about her hobby or realized that it was simply a spasm from her favorite activity. Horse riding is a hobby, a joy, a pastime, therapeutic even and, in her case, a perpetuating factor for a crippling back condition. Two deep tissue treatments and she was restored to full health, back to her horses and her smile was now genuine. I love my job!

Understanding how the accident happened can create a visual understanding, or mental tableau, of what may have happened to your client's body at the moment of trauma. If you can visualize how and where they were sitting, where they were looking at the moment of impact, where the car struck their vehicle, and what they felt on impact, you can actually create an empathetic understanding of the injuries from which client is likely suffering. What do you do with that information? You palpate and treat every associated muscular structure that may be affected. You will usually surprise yourself with how helpful this is.

Latin and Soup

If a patient walked into the average doctor's office with a knife stuck in their head, the doctor would do two things. First, they would name their pain in Latin. "Ah, you have 'Knifus Cranius!'" The thought probably sounds absurd, but it is true. Doctors have told me that their patients feel as though they were robbed if the doctor cannot give them a name for their pain and a drug prescription to take care of the problem.

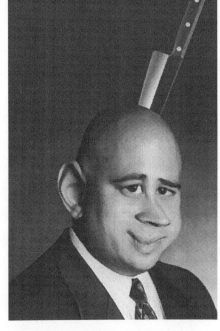

A few years back, as I talked with my family physician during my annual physical, I shared a laugh with him about the absurdity of that mindset. He said, "How did you know we do that?!"

A severe case of "Knifus Cranius."

"I see it all the time. A patient tells you that their tissues hurt, and you translate what they just said in Latin: Fibromyalgia. When my daughters are being stubborn, I tell them they have a severe case of 'gluteal myalgia'." In plain English that means, pain in the butt.

He laughed. "Okay, since you know that's what we do,

I have a story to tell you," he said. "I had a patient who came in saying her anus itched. I gave her a prescription for cortisone cream and told her she had "pruritus ani." When she went home that night to meet a friend for drinks, the friend asked what she had done that day. My patient said she had seen her doctor for treatment of pruritus ani and her friend choked on her drink. 'Your doctor said your butt itches, but he said it in Latin. *I* speak Latin. I wouldn't spread that diagnosis around.'"

I still laugh about that story.

The point is, it is not so much the diagnosis that is important, but the cure.

When a patient sees a medical doctor after a car accident, they get two things. One, they are given a name for their pain, such as "cervical sprain and strain" or "whiplash." Then, they get what I call, "The Soup," a cocktail of drugs that includes muscle relaxants, painkillers and anti-inflammatories. They *always* get the soup. The trouble is, the longer that they stay on the drugs and wait to receive therapy, the longer it will take for them to get well.

In addition to "The Soup," they will often also have to deal with something called "Narcotic Withdrawal Syndrome," after they have been on narcotic painkillers for an extended period of time. I could write an entire book about Narcotic Withdrawal Syndrome, but instead, I will devote an entire chapter to it, later in this book. It is important to understand as a healthcare practitioner and that includes massage therapists.

Scar Tissue and Timeframes

Given the opportunity, I would love to begin treatment with a client on the day of an automobile collision. A friend once said to me, "If I could, I would reach my hands in the window at the scene of an accident to begin treatment." I fully agree.

But, what were you told in school? How long were you told to wait before treating a client who had just been struck by a car? A week? Two? Six-weeks? Every moment that passes, after a collision, gives scar tissue a chance to continue building in the body. Scar tissue, or collagen, is sticky stuff. I usually refer to scar tissue as "Biblical", because scar tissue "begets" scar tissue -it just keeps on laying down.

It has been taught that if you rub scar tissue with "cross fiber friction, "you can make it go away. Not true. Scar tissue is sticky stuff and a lot like chewing gum.

If you had gum in your hair and I massaged it and rubbed it, would it go away? Probablynot. It would get warmer, softer, and more pliable, but it would not go away. Rubbing it does "break it up," but it stays put. If we want to make it go away, our only real option is to change it.

Just how do you change scar tissue and what are the benefits of "changing" it? Simple. When scar tissue has been adequately worked and is pliable, you are better able to stretch the muscle fibers that are involved. This forces the fibers of the scar tissue to "come along for the ride," and stretches them into position alongside the muscle tissue.

When those fibers lay alongside each other, the brain gets "tricked" into believing that the scar tissue is actually muscle tissue. The result is increased tensile strength and elasticity. That change stops the body from laying down more scar tissue. It is easy to prove. As scar and fascial tissues are stretched after being warmed, they become more malleable. Stretching them, along with the associated muscle, forces those tissues to comply and follow the lead of the stretch. Now, rather than fighting the direction of the scar tissue, the tissues now work *with* the client and the body reacts favorably as a result.

There is another important aspect that you should keep in mind when it comes to scar tissue: It is a lot like turkey soup in the refrigerator. Let me explain.

After Thanksgiving every year, my father makes his amazing, turkey soup. As he has been getting along in years, he has slowly passed that tradition on to me, but the memories of his magic touch will live on forever in the minds of the Haase clan as we anticipate his next batch.

To make the soup, he tosses the leftover meat and turkey bones into a big stockpot, fills it with water and lets it simmer for an entire day. After he has turned off the burner and it begins to cool, he places it in our refrigerator and allows it to completely cool overnight. The next morning, all of the fat congeals into a hard, flat disk that floats on the top, allowing it to be easily removed. Nearly fat-free soup! Why am I talking about soup in a massage book? Because that "fat disk" helps make my point.

You see, that molten turkey fat has a lot in common with our fascia and scar tissue. When you ice fascia and scar tissue, it hardens. After you perform cross-fiber friction on a client's scar tissue, it warms and becomes more malleable. Next, you stretch those fibers, allowing them to migrate into the same linear direction as the muscle tissue. It is only *then* that you ice it. If you ice prior to the stretch, you risk further irritation of the scar tissue formation process because cold fibers do not stretch well.

You may have been taught to have your plantar fasciitis clients freeze a bottle of water at home and then have them roll their foot over the bottle in order to cool the plantar fasciitis inflammation. It *is* a great technique. That said, it is a bad technique if your client rolls their foot over the bottle, which shortens the fibers on the sole of the foot and makes those fibers harden, and then they stand on them right away. That first step will literally rip away at the already distressed tissues and exacerbate the condition.

If you recommend this "frozen bottle icing technique", be sure to tell your clients to make it the very last thing that they do before going to bed at night. Have them sit on the edge of the bed, roll their foot on the ice bottle, then lie back in bed and not get up for at least 30-minutes. This will give the foot's plantar tissues a chance to return to normal temperature and minimize the chance of exacerbation.

Limited Evaluation

A lot of massage therapists get caught up in the intricacies of muscle testing, and for good reason. They were taught how to test in school. My problem with the whole idea of muscle testing is twofold.

One, it has been shown in numerous studies that even physical therapists and medical doctors have been wrong when testing for injuries. They have obtained false positives as well as false negatives with their testing.

My second issue is that we are massage therapists and are not allowed to make a diagnosis. Yes, many therapists skirt the "diagnosis" issue by saying that they are "assessing" the client, but the truth is, most are actually diagnosing.

If a doctor sends their patient to you with a script that says the patient has a specific condition, we must treat for that. However, if we have a client looking for answers as to why they are in pain, they want to know what you are finding. This is dangerous territory. You can say, "The muscles of the right rotator cuff appear injured and I am going to try some techniques to diminish your pain while increasing your function." What you cannot say is, "You have a torn rotator cuff muscle."

Most massage clients will tell you that they prefer going to a massage therapist who spends the session performing massage rather than testing.

The therapist who performs test after test just makes the client even more frustrated. "Does this hurt? Does this hurt? Does it hurt when you resist this? How about this? Does this hurt?" All they hear are a lot questions when what they really want to hear are some answers about how to improve their health.

Clients want to be massaged and your testing can actually exacerbate the condition (keep in mind the section about "the less a muscle is touched..."). Not good, especially if you are aggravating your client with your incessant muscle tests.

There is good news though. Are you ready? Here it is: "If it hurts, squish it." I still laugh when I think about the first time I heard that phrase.

Back in the early 1990's, I took a workshop from a naturopathic physician. She had the skills of a naturopath, chiropractor and massage therapist all wrapped up into one. As she was working on a student's neck during a demonstration, I asked, "What muscle are you working on?"

She lifted her head, scrunched her face up and said, "I don't know! If it hurts, squish it!"

Simple philosophy, isn't it? Sure, she probably knew the name of the muscle, but what she conveyed was the bigger picture. Work on muscles that are in pain. Pain is an indicator. Muscles without pain likely do not have any issues since healthy tissues should not feel pain when palpated with moderate pressure.

Your shoulder, for example, has four muscles that hold the humerus to the shoulder girdle. If one of them hurts while you massage it, it *needs* massage. Not really a complicated process, is it? While you can spend your time testing the shoulder with the dozens of shoulder tests available to you, I think your client would be more impressed that you found and relieved their pain. If it hurts, squish it!

Understanding Injury

Prior to treatment, it is important to understand just how the injury took place and what the conditions were prior to and during the injury.

During my early days at the athletic club, I had a married couple that would receive massage from me on a regular basis. The wife came in weekly. She was an amazing athlete. On a *weekly* basis, she would do aerobics, racquetball, scuba diving, tennis, weights, dirt bike riding, and bicycling. Every massage was for the purpose of keeping her active. With deep, consistent work, I helped her accomplish that goal and her muscles were an amazing example of healthy tissue. Her husband, however, received just two massages a year. Is that considered regular? Yes, but unfortunately it was not as often as what he needed.

He was an attorney who spent most of his days at his desk so he was not nearly as active, or healthy, as his wife.

One summer, the two were on vacation in Hawaii. Since they were avid motorcycle riders, they rented a Harley-Davidson Road King and toured the Island of Maui. One fateful afternoon, they were waiting at a stop light and were hit by a semi-truck driver who was lost. He had been looking down at a map while traveling at 50+ miles per hour. Not only did he not see the red light, but he also did not see the couple on their motorcycle.

At the moment of impact, both were thrown a significant distance and landed on the pavement far in front of the point of impact. It was not pretty. But miraculously, there were no broken bones, just soft tissue injuries.

In the end, she needed only four treatments, over a two-week period, to restore her muscles to her pre-injury state. However, her husband required numerous treatments over a six-month period. The difference was that her muscles were in amazing shape from frequent treatment and activity prior to the collision while her husband's were not.

Children have a huge advantage when it comes to recovery from soft tissue injuries compared to those out of their teen years. They have resilient tissues with bodies built for repair whereas adults increasingly lose more of their regeneration ability with each passing year. Understanding the age relationship to healing will help in your treatment strategies.

Perpetuating Factors

For the massage therapist who addresses injuries, understanding perpetuating factors of injury and pain is one of the most important aspects of care that you can address.

Let us address the knife in the head, or "Knifus Cranius." The knife is the perpetuating factor. The wound is the injury. We can massage around the knife, medicate the patient for pain, clean around the knife to prevent infection, but until you remove that knife, even the best of care is useless.

The same is true for your clients. If they have work, home or lifestyle conditions that are keeping them in an injured or physiologically aggravated state, the best massage and myotherapy in the world cannot return them to health and physiological homeostasis. That is, they will not *stay* that way for very long. The client will go right back to his old habits and the condition will return.

Early in my practice, I met a gentleman who had been hurt on the job and needed to be completely ambulatory before he would be allowed to return to work. On his first day of treatment, he arrived in a wheel chair. As he improved with my treatments, he graduated to a walker, crutches, and then a cane. But we were both frustrated that he was not completely better and able to toss the cane once and for all. That is when my true understanding of the importance of a thorough "perpetuating factor interview" began.

I asked him a series of questions. Since he was not really driving anywhere and was staying mostly at home, it did not take long to get to the true culprit.

"What do you spend your days doing?

"Uh... you know... stuff."

"Stuff like what?"

"You know, odds and ends."

He fidgeted. For a man who got his hands dirty for a living and had lived a productive life of physical labor, it was apparent that something made him uncomfortable about my line of questioning.

"Describe your average day. What did you do yesterday?"

"Well, I got up, showered, had breakfast, and then watched TV."

"That's it?

"Well, I had lunch and dinner too."

"And the rest of the time?"

"Uh..."

"I need you to come clean with me. Are you watching TV from after breakfast until you go to bed?"

He looked down. "Yeah, I guess so. I actually watch it during meals too."

"I need you to do something for me. I want you to continue watching TV just as you have been, but every 15-minutes, I want you to grab your cane and walk around your house twice. Then you can go back to sitting in your "Lazy Boy" (which is ironically named) and watch TV."

Mind you, this was in the days before Tivo, so he could not pause shows and ensure he did not miss anything. Even so, I was able to get Steven to commit to his, four-times-an-hour, double-trip around his house. Then I told him not to come back to see me for 7-days.

When Steven returned 7-days later, he was beaming.

"Notice I'm not using a cane? I get to go back to work!"

It was after that experience that I did not take on the, frustration and responsibility of getting my clients better.

Early on in my career I learned this cornerstone on which to build your own massage practice. Movement is Life, Lack of Movement is Death... get your clients moving!

Americans readily spend money on their houses, vacations, cars, jewelry and electronics, but skimp where we spend most of our time: a good bed, pillow, vehicle seat, office chair, living room recliner and shoes. We tend to make excuses for not investing in what is important, or only buy mattresses because they were on sale. We will not take care of our back and use our own money to buy ourselves our own office chair because it is the "company's responsibility" to do that. We wear flip-flops or other shoes because they are "cute" rather than purchase shoes than ensure our posture and health.

More often than not, your clients have life habits or activities that continue them on a path of stagnation, exacerbation and degeneration. Even though we are not occupational therapists, we do have the ability to ask questions and give suggestions for our clients to alter their workspaces and lifestyle habits.

Let's discuss the questions that I usually ask my clients who seem to be unable to get well and/or inhibited in their healing process.

Perpetuating Factors: Work

What do you do for a living? Is it a repetitive task? Describe your workstation. Where is your keyboard? Monitor? Are you required to lift loads? What weights?

Years ago, I visited a local bank to cash a check which I had received. When I entered, it was clear that the bank had remodeled since I was last there. The high, teller counters were gone and replaced with beautiful, cherry wood desks. The eye-level monitors which the tellers used were now dropped below a glass platen on the desk surface. Teller keyboards were lower as well.

As I made small talk with the teller, I asked her when the remodel was complete and she said it was complete a month earlier. "Isn't it so beautiful in here now?" she asked.

"It's really nice. How are your headaches doing?"

With a look of disbelief and her eyes wide, she asked, "How on earth did you know I had a headache?"

I wanted to have a little fun with her so I touched my forehead with the back of my hand, like a cheesy mentalist in a carnival, and closed my eyes. I followed up with, "The headache... it's at the base of your skull..."

She gasped. "You're good!"

I strained harder, in deep concentration... "You've had it for about a month..."

"Oh my goodness! How do you *do* that?!"

I cracked a big smile and opened my eyes. "Ma'am...

your bank remodeled recently, moving your monitor so that you now have to crane your neck down, and you've been doing that for a month." I smirked as it sank in.

Coincidentally, the bank fixed the problem later that year. Apparently it was a better option than paying higher worker's compensation insurance premiums for their injured workers.

I still do not comprehend the number of people who use their shoulder to hold their phone to their ear and then complain, "Man, my neck really hurts." Nearly every type of phone has a hands-free option of some sort. At my seminar headquarters, I use a simple $10.00 Panasonic headset with boom-microphone that allows me to talk and use my hands at the same time. That is a tiny price to pay for the prevention of neck pain.

As a side note, if you do use a wireless "Bluetooth" type of headset or earpiece, be sure to keep the phone off and away from your body. According to research by The National University of Cuyo in Argentina, it has been determined that men who typically wear their cell phones on their right hips have a reduced level of bone minerals and bone density in the area of the right hip, but not the left. Similar results were also revealed by Turkish researchers at the Suleyman Demirel University in Isparta.

Bones break down and rebuild as a part of our body's natural maintenance, however it appears that the radiation from cell phones is altering that rebuilding process.

Just a thought, but you also might want to consider where you keep your phone. My daughters like to use their bra as a phone holder and I am doing my best to convince them to alter that habit. If it is affecting bone growth and metabolism, it may have more impact on other tissues as well. Of course, the cell companies do not concur, but time will tell.

Perpetuating Factors: Transportation

What kind of vehicle do you drive? Is the seat supportive of your lumbar region? Does the height allow your pelvis proper position? Is it a manual or automatic transmission? How many hours do you drive a day? Where do you position your arms/hands while driving?

Years ago I purchased a shiny, new Volkswagen Jetta. It was an awesome car. I did not realize it when I bought it, but my foot did not really fit in the foot-well and I had to tilt it at a 45-degree angle in order to use the gas pedal. I really did not notice the pain that started to build in my right hip and gluteal area until a month after I bought the car. I looked down at my feet and, sure enough, my left foot pointed directly ahead and my right foot was turned at a 45-degree angle. My car was causing me issues and I needed a new one! Once I did, all was better. Although I had been receiving great massage on my deep lateral rotators, the pain would not resolve until I dealt with the perpetuating factor of my car's insufficient foot-well.

Amidst my pain, I laughed out loud at my predicament. One of my mentors once said that if both feet point outwards from tight external rotators, you have "lawyer's ass." I figured I must have "legal assistant's ass" since only one foot was pointing outwards.

I had a woman that was seeing me for treatment of her left hip and leg. I could actually see that the left leg was developing more muscle mass compared to the right leg and it was affecting her quality of life. After I continued to ask questions about her life, she mentioned that her leg bothered her the most while she drove her "stick-shift" Chevy Nova. A few months prior to seeking treatment, she had gotten a "special deal" on a replacement spring for her clutch pedal. It was for a big truck, but it fit. When we had it tested, we found it took three times the normal pressure to depress the pedal! The poor woman spent significant hours in her car each day. Essentially she was doing one-legged exercises all day long, which over –worked the muscles and brought imbalance to her legs and hip. Once the clutch spring was corrected, her symptoms began to improve.

Perpetuating Factors: Sleep

How many hours do you usually sleep a night? What type of pillow do you use? How many pillows do you use? Do you use bolsters or body pillows for support? Do you sleep on your back, side, or belly? What type of mattress do you have? How old is it?

The number of clients who have come into my office with "sleep injuries" is stunning to me. Usually the first words out of their mouths are, "I slept funky last night." My first question is, "Were you drinking prior to going to bed?" The answer is, "yes," more often than not. We tend to not feel any pain when we are inebriated and can easily sleep like a contortionist without realizing it – at least until we wake up with a "funky" pain.

Even without alcohol, most people do not realize how a poor quality mattress and/or pillow can be a detriment to their sleep posture. We as therapists need to discuss sleep posture, as well as bolstering, with every one of our clients.

Sleep Tips:

- The best "pillow" is actually a small, rolled-up towel held in place with a couple of rubber bands. This allows the client to sleep on their back or side while supporting the neck's natural kyphotic curve.

- Side-sleepers need a pillow under their top leg to keep the knee from dropping all the way down to the bed. This reduces the stress on the hip joint and associated muscles. People with wider hips are especially affected by side sleeping as hip width increases the distance the knee drops to the bed surface.

- Belly sleepers are a difficult bunch. Telling someone to change his or her position, after a lifetime habit has been formed, is nearly impossible. If the client does sleep on their belly, at least have them put a small pillow under the shoulder/chest on the side their head is facing toward. This will keep the horizontal rotation of the neck from reaching its end-feel and reduce tension.

Interestingly, I have found that belly sleepers find comfort in the pressure that they sense against their stomach and chest from the mattress. If the client's neck is being significantly compromised, you may want to suggest a "weighted blanket" to cover them as they go to sleep in a supine position. The weight seems to bring comfort, allowing them to drift off to sleep. The emotional and psychological benefits also appear to be significant from my observations.

Perpetuating Factors: Home

What do you do when you get home after work? How do you spend your days off at home? How do you spend your evenings? What kind of chair do you sit on?

You would be surprised to learn how most of your clients spend their after-work/evening hours. After laying in bed all night, then sitting in their office chair all day, they grab a six-pack of beer and sit in their favorite chair to watch television until it is time to repeat the cycle.

Many of our clients have hyperkyphosis not because of bad posture, but because they are creating it with self-induced "molds." They sleep on an old mattress that has too much sag or support their heads with extra pillows, which contributes to exaggerated curves. Again, they often have poor office chairs, non-supportive vehicle seats and poorly designed lounge chairs which lack postural support.

My parents spent a good deal of money on a very nice, leather, dual-recliner sofa in which they sat to watch TV. It had a great, built-in, head pillow- rest and looked really nice. I watched my mother sitting in it and the source of her recent postural changes became obvious. The back "support" was not supportive and the headrest actually pushed her head forward. She literally sank into the chair while her neck was forced into flexion. She had to use the recliner function, which tilted her torso back, in order to lift her eyes enough to comfortably see the television. It was not until my parents replaced that love seat that her posture was corrected. My parents are not the only ones who have had to deal with "nice looking furniture" that created or exacerbated postural distortions.

Perpetuating Factors: Legs & Feet

What kind of shoes do you wear? How many different shoes do you wear each week? What is the wear pattern on the bottom of your shoes? Do you wear orthotics? Are you aware of any leg length discrepancies?

While it is outside the scope of practice for a massage therapist to diagnose true leg length discrepancies, knowing the discrepancy exists is imperative to our ability to help our clients recover.

When a chiropractor says, "Your legs are different lengths... let me fix that," they are not actually going to put your short leg into a leg stretcher. They are referring to a rotation in the pelvis that makes the leg *appear* shorter. Anatomical length and actual physiological length are two different things. A femur that is even 5mm shorter will have a direct pathological impact on the body, forcing it to adapt. That adaptation can take many different directions such as scoliosis or TMJD issues. If there is a bone length discrepancy, it needs to be addressed before you can truly make a difference. Palliative care will be of benefit, but not with any form of lasting result.

If a client has the length addressed via a shoe shim, it is imperative that the shim height be *gradually* added over a period of days or weeks to allow the body to adapt. If the length is changed all at once, the body will usually react adversely.

I would never presume to tell a chiropractor that they are wrong, but I am adamantly opposed to one leg-length correction method that has been used by chiropractors for many years, called a "heel lift." If the leg is truly short on one side, you need to lift the entire foot, not just the heel.

Try it for yourself. Stand up and exaggeratedly lift your right heel off of the ground. What happens to your hips? They rotate. Heel lifts may make your client feel good for a short while, but the body's attempt to adapt to the rotation brings even more trouble. Good for increased business for the doctor, bad for the client's health.

During my seminars, I am frequently asked my opinion regarding the barefoot running movement and minimalist running shoes. I do agree that the increased foot movement encourages foot health. However, the idea is flawed, unless you are talking about running on soft surfaces.

Our feet and bodies are not designed for the hard, flat surfaces in our man-made environment. The reason we need orthotics in our shoes is to adapt to the "flatness" of the world and most of us need them for optimal health.

If you truly want to get your feet healthy, I have a

suggestion for your massage room, or better yet, your entire home. If you were to make all your floors into a 6" deep sandbox, then force all of your visiting friends, family and clients to walk barefoot on sand versus hard floors, you would do them a world of good. Granted, it would be difficult to clean, but it would let our feet function as they were intended. If we were born with flat feet, then flat floors would be perfect. Since that is not the case, you have two options... either make your feet able to adapt to the surface, or have a surface that can adapt to your feet.

One last note about leg-length discrepancies. If a client with equal leg lengths has a straight spine while standing, but a scoliotic curvature while sitting, then they may be dealing with a "small hemi-pelvis." A small hemi-pelvis is where one ilium is smaller than the other and causes the ischial tuberosity to drop down to meet the sitting surface. It causes the hips to drop on one side and brings a lateral curve to the spine. Most people who are dealing with this condition usually have an urge to always cross their legs in order to adapt to the imbalance. It is a tell-tale sign and the first question I ask if I suspect a small hemi-pelvis.

You cannot diagnose this, but you can observe it and suggest modifications to your client's posture and work environment. To do this, have your client expose their back and sit on a hard, flat bench while you observe them from behind. Notice the spinous processes. If the processes curve laterally while sitting, but are more vertical while standing, then a small hemi-pelvis is likely present. You can experiment by placing magazines beneath the lower side until the spine appears straight. This "butt shim" should actually make the client feel more comfortable as they sit with the shim in place. Note the total thickness of the magazines once you find that "sweet spot" on the spine. The client can now use this information to place a shim under their lower side at work or while sitting at home or in the car.

Perpetuating Factors: Diet

How much water do you drink? Are you taking supplements? What kind? How much? Do you eat whole, raw foods or mostly processed foods?

Recommending or suggesting vitamins, minerals or the like is a very gray area for massage therapists. We do not have the client's complete medical history, therefore we are not aware of potential contraindications or complications such as mixing certain vitamins with a heart medication that the doctor prescribed for the patient. Not to mention, prescribing is outside of our scope of practice.

Educating your clients about the *value* of certain supplements can be helpful, but make sure you say, "Please be sure to ask your doctor before taking a supplement... I can't prescribe, just tell you what others have found to be helpful..."

For example, I recommend that clients take a high quality, easily absorbable calcium supplement if they are dealing with muscular contraction issues. Muscle cells need calcium ions to function, but that is another book in and of itself. I can say, "My athletes, who have night cramps in their calf muscles, seem to do better and stop the cramps if they take at least 1,500mg of calcium before they go to bed at night, but you may to want to ask your dietitian or family doctor first." You cannot tell your client, however, that they should take four Mezotrace brand mineral tablets every evening, prior to bed. That is *prescribing*. Too gray? It can be a fine line, but educating your clients about the basics of good nutrition and encouraging them to seek the advice of a nutritional consultant is encouraged.

Most massage therapists suggest that their clients drink water after their massage and with good reason. There are many health benefits to hydrating tissues after a massage, and beforehand as well, for that matter. Understanding your client's hydration habits and encouraging them is paramount for tissue recovery. It also helps to explain to your clients about how beef jerky is made. Even filet mignon can become beef jerky if you remove the moisture.

Here is the logic. If your client breathes on a mirror, they see moisture. With every breath, with every blink of the eye, with every breeze over our skin, we lose moisture. Life, by its very nature is a "human dehydrator" and we evaporate with every moment. Our bodies are mostly water and *lack of* water replacement can cause a boatload of troubles, including decreased brain function, decreased blood production and the loss of function with our muscles as well. Suggesting that your clients need water is more than okay. Educate and give them a bottle for the road!

Since the term "diet" has to do with purposeful consumption of nutrients and substances through the mouth, this is a good place to discuss cigarette smoking.

I have found that cigarette smokers have a difficult

time fully recovering from their aches and pains and it is directly due to the smoke. Trying to get a smoker to quit can be difficult, but I figured out a way to increase your odds of success. It will not make any friends, but it just may save a life.

Realize that telling a client that they may die from smoking is about as effective as telling an 18-year old that they should save their money for retirement. They cannot see the immediate benefit, so they ignore your suggestion. With that in mind, this is how I discuss the issue with smokers...

"Mr. Stanton, I can't treat you anymore."

"Why?"

"Well, you're robbing the insurance company that is paying for your massage and I can't ethically support that."

"What are you talking about??"

"Let me see if I can help you understand... Let's say a man knocked on my office door right now with a hammer in his hand. As I open the door, he smacks himself in the head and then says, 'I have a headache. Can you get rid of my headache?' And then he hits himself in the head again! You would think he is crazy, right? You'd take him to the mental hospital and tell them to take good care of the crazy man."

"What does that have to do with me?"

"Well, Mr. Stanton, you have this little bus driver in your blood called hemoglobin. That bus driver is a bigot. It loves carbon monoxide, but despises oxygen. When both are on the curb, waiting their turn to get on the bus, the driver lets the carbon monoxide on first and whatever space is left goes to the oxygen. For your muscles to function properly, they need oxygen. The presence of carbon monoxide diminishes that oxygen and increases your spasm.

"Mr. Stanton, that spasm presents to your brain as stress and you say you smoke to decrease the stress. You are stressed because you smoke and you smoke because you're stressed. *You* are the cause of your pain, but you want me to bill your insurance company and to alleviate the pain that you are purposely causing. You might as well just hit your head with a hammer."

"I... I can't just stop smoking."

"Mr. Stanton, how much do you smoke?"

"Two packs a day."

"Okay... look, it takes 24-hours for carbon monoxide to clear your system. Here is what I want you to do. I want you to smoke four packs of cigarettes, every other day, between 8:00am and 9:00am. You can get all of your cigarette smoking in, but give your muscles a chance to clear and reduce your stress levels."

"I can't do that!"

"Then maybe you should find a way to quit, because the cigarette you smoke today is causing the pain you are feeling today. If you do not care that you are killing yourself slowly, that's your decision, but you are causing your pain. Your choices. Your pain. Your decision."

It might sound harsh, but I have had this conversation hundreds of times over the years. Once I help a client understand that they are causing their own pain, they sometimes make a decision to quit.

Perpetuating Factors: Pain Management Medications

Narcotic Withdrawal Syndrome

I want to be clear about my beliefs regarding painkillers. I do not believe it is humane to allow anyone to suffer if there is a valid option to decrease suffering. For people in pain, medication can give them their lives back and allow them to function on a daily basis. However, if the pain medication is not managed and taken properly, the results can be devastating. This chapter is about understanding the effects of long-term use of opiates and how that affects your clients.

During my seminars, I always give an opportunity for students to ask me questions about any topic. Invariably, I get questions as to my opinion about the use of narcotics, painkillers and medical marijuana for patients with pain.

The use of narcotics-opiates is not always a negative thing. The problems seem to result from over-prescribing of these medications, as well as the consequences of the long-term effects. Studies show that narcotic painkillers are linked to a variety of dangerous side effects including sharply reduced hormone production, sleep apnea, increased falls and hip fractures in the elderly and, in extreme cases, fatal overdoses.

In 2011, Washington State took the strongest stance yet regarding the over-prescribing of opioids, including hydrocodone, fentanyl, methadone and oxycodone (the active ingredient in OxyContin). The doctor must now refer the patient to a pain specialist for evaluation if the underlying condition is not improving.

Sadly, out of fear of retribution from the government, many doctors are refusing to treat patients who need pain medicines and many patients are finding that their current doctors are refusing to refill prescriptions as they had done in the past. Many who really need the medications are suffering needlessly.

While medications should be available to help patients cope with pain, the doctors must also actively be working to help the patient deal with the underlying cause of the pain. Writing a script is easy and quick, whereas researching and creating a treatment plan takes more work. With so many doctors dealing with lower payment reimbursement from insurance companies and their patient rosters splitting at the seams, it is easy to understand why doctors take the quicker route. The idea of using opioids for long term pain relief is relatively new, with increased use in the past 15-years or so. As doctors found that patients were getting long-term relief, all seemed well. But as tolerance increased, so did the prescribed dosages and subsequent side effects, such as death. While doctors should be monitoring the patient's care and response to the medications, few have time to do so and things have gotten out of control.

For chronic pain, research has shown that opiates usually tend to make pain worse, causing the client to need larger and larger doses. In some cases, the use of narcotics can actually *cause* pain. Not only does the patient suffer more pain, but now they also have to deal with the plethora of side effects from taking the drugs.

Taking narcotics inhibits the body's ability to make endorphins, its own natural painkillers. Endorphins increase during sleep and while performing aerobic exercise, but decrease from lack of sleep and the use of narcotics. They can also interfere with the ability to think with clarity, which ultimately affects job performance.

Over time, narcotics can make nerves more sensitive, making the pain even worse. Narcotics can also slow the bowel and lead to constipation, bloating, nausea and difficulty urinating.

Another, more specific, problem is called Narcotic Bowel Syndrome, or NBS. The syndrome is not always recognized but is becoming more common from the chronic use of narcotic painkillers. The syndrome involves chronic or intermittent abdominal pain that gets increasingly worse as the effect of the drug diminishes. In addition to the pain, those with NBS may experience bloating, periodic vomiting, nausea, constipation and abdominal distention.

What is most relevant for massage therapists to understand are the dynamics of what is referred to as Narcotic Withdrawal Syndrome. Although massage therapists obviously cannot diagnose, prescribe, or get involved with the client's medication regimen, the therapist *can* be a part of educating and helping the client understand how specific medications are affecting the recovery process.

So what are the effects on the client from taking pain medications, especially for an extended period of time? One of the biggest issues to understand is that physical neglect of the body intensifies pain. At the same time, lack of use or overuse can decrease tissue health. Pain medications lead to both.

When a client is on opiates to reduce pain, they often feel a decrease in desire to do much at all in the way of physical activity, which results in a reduction in their state of health. Again, Movement is Life, Lack of Movement is Death. Lack of movement leads to muscle atrophy. Pain medications have a large role to play in this because the client often feels numb, lacks energy because they feel sleepy, or lifeless and devoid of motivation.

The reverse of this is also true for some patients under the influence of pain medications. If they cannot really feel the pain, clients end up overtaxing their bodies and push beyond normal pain barriers. Where the average person would say, "Hey, this really hurts I should back off and not continue what I'm doing," the person being numbed by opiates receives no such feedback. They overuse the muscles and exacerbate injury to their body in the process.

People addicted to narcotic painkillers often believe they need more of the drug because their pain is getting worse. That pain can be from the overuse of the drug and lack of direct pain feedback or from lack of exercise because they feel lethargic.

Another way that the pain medications can worsen the client's health is from poor posture. When the patient feels no pain or discomfort from abnormal positioning, the body cannot make the needed self-corrections. This results in a perpetuation of pain. Much like the client who goes to bed drunk, sleeps in a catawampus position and then wakes up with neck strain. The pain-medicated client ends up with the same result for similar reasons. The client's poor posture is directly related to lack of sensation which allows for positions that they normally would not find comfortable. Instead of correcting the position or habits that lead to increased pain, the client just takes more painkillers. It is a vicious cycle of physical neglect that is concealed by the drugs themselves.

What is misunderstood by most people who regularly consume opiate-based painkillers are the dynamics of withdrawal. Most believe that "quitting" a drug means they have stopped taking it for good. The truth is, every time the drug begins to wear off, there is an experience of withdrawal, which is beyond unpleasant.

The between-dosages withdrawal that occurs often feels like an intensification of the very symptoms which the person was trying to escape through taking the painkillers in the first place. In other words, the withdrawal magnifies the original pain until you feed it more of the drug. Shortly after the client takes the next dose of the drug, the unpleasant withdrawal symptoms stop and the person feels the pain disappear. This offers temporary relief, relaxation, decreased tension and emotional distress – until the next dose is due.

It may sound like I am implying that the drug itself is sentient, or has a mind of its own. That thought has more truth to it than you realize. I had a client that went off of pain meds in the setting of a 28-day rehab facility. She experienced not only a spike of the original pain for which she was medicating, but also re-experienced pain from injuries that she had sustained during her childhood, youth and young adulthood. The pains increased and were relentless. The withdrawal was excruciating until she finally reclaimed her body as her own again.

The experience of coming off of pain meds is said to be nearly synonymous with an exorcism. Whether it is stopping for just a few hours or for days on end, the pain will increase due to withdrawal pains, until the ugly monster is either fed what it desires or starved to death once and for all. Do not underestimate the power of opiates to affect your clients in ways you may have never thought possible. And beware. Some people will stop at nothing to get their hands on more. Our prisons are full of those who did not survive the withdrawal process.

If your client decides to get off of opiates, they need to first realize that their dependency on the pain medication can often intensify the pain, making it difficult to determine which pain is from the original injury and which is from the use of the narcotics.

This is the most important aspect of the detoxification from opiate narcotics. Most patients have the same level or less pain *after* detoxification. Seriously, read that again. *Most* patients have no difference in pain levels or have even *less* pain after they get the drugs out of their systems. Sure, it takes an agonizing month for their body to get clean, but once they have completed their detox, their bodies will usually feel better than they did before detox.

If your patient or client is going to get off of narcotics, such as long-acting morphine, OxyContin, hydrocodone, Tylenol #3, Codeine, Darvocet, Percodan and the like, they need to do so under the guidance of their doctor. In all reality, they really should do so under direct supervision in a rehab facility. Quitting all at once may actually result in death.

Marijuana

Although I do not use medical marijuana myself, I believe it is an excellent option for those who could reap the benefits of its use. Sadly, our government has done an excellent job of vilifying the use of this natural plant that grows wild throughout the world. The government does not mention that endogenous cannabinoids are naturally produced in the human body.

Science demonstrates that cannabinoid receptor activation is a natural and important component for proper, early development in humans. As a matter of fact, there is a hormone in human breast milk that activates the receptor sites for cannabinoids. If that receptor site development is disrupted, it can have catastrophic effects, including disrupting feeding behavior. Studies have shown that if a drug is introduced to rats that blocks cannabinoid receptors, half of the rats will die.

Am I saying that we should all smoke pot? No. I am saying that it is probably the most natural of all available painkillers on the market, right next to good old aspirin. While our government approves the use of toxic chemicals like acetaminophen (proven by their own manufactures to damage our livers), it wants to block a natural herb that functions efficiently in our bodies for a variety of ailments.

The very politicians that want its use blocked stand around at political fundraisers, with a glass of alcohol in hand, and discuss how "pot" is a bad drug. Really? I believe that we either need to outlaw alcohol, or make marijuana legal. It is not that difficult to look at the ridiculous logic. While millions of Americans are guilty of drinking and driving every year, most pot smokers prefer to stay home and eat some snacks before drifting off asleep. Overuse of alcohol has more damaging effects to the body compared with very few known, adverse affects from the overuse of pot.

A police officer told me, off the record, that he would much rather deal with a pot-smoking driver, heading down the freeway at 35-miles per hour while playing Bob Marley music than a drunk driver who was speeding and swerving fearlessly amongst unsuspecting drivers and pedestrians.

There. I have said my peace. While I do not "enjoy the benefits" of marijuana myself, I believe the option should be available to those who would benefit from its use.

Unveiling Myths, Misnomers and Misinformation

Cancer

During massage school, I was told, "massage on a cancer patient is contraindicated because we can spread the cancer." Years later, it became clear that massage is generally *good* for the cancer patient. However it is dependant on the individual condition and/or treatment protocol. So, why did the general consensus regarding massage and cancer patients change? It is not so much about why it is suddenly okay to massage cancer patients, but about the reasons why it was not okay in the first place. As massage therapists, we must know why we should or should not perform a technique with every client. It always comes back to the simple question of "why?"

As a Renegade Massage Therapist, you need to ask questions and use common sense, especially regarding the issue of massaging cancer patients. First of all, I am a great massage therapist, but I am not so good that I can change someone's DNA or cellular issues, leading to cancer running rampant. Cancer is ultimately a "DNA thing" or a cellular "miscommunication" problem, and therefore massage cannot directly affect that. That said, could I put a tumor at risk by applying direct pressure or break a bone that is compromised due to the effects of radiation or chemotherapy? Absolutely. Can cancer spread because of massage? No. The heart affects circulation far more than your massage will.

Here is the simple logic of why we are now told that it is okay to massage a cancer patient, barring specific conditions that may prelude treatment:

- Doctors said "no" to the patient when it came to receiving massage, but "yes" to exercise.

- Exercise increases circulation.
- Massage increases circulation.
- Exercise boosts the immune system and increases quality of life.
- Massage boosts the immune system and increases quality of life.
- Simple math. If A equals B, and B equals C, then A equals C, meaning massage is a benefit, not a hazard.

With that realization, Memorial Sloan-Kettering Hospital in New York City was one of the first in the nation to begin offering massage, and other "complimentary" care to its patients, with great acceptance. Even better, one single massage could alleviate nausea for a couple of days versus a nausea medication that costs in excess of $200.00 per pill.

Sometimes, while working with an attending physician, it is *how* you approach them as you ask about offering massage. A doctor once said, "Absolutely not!" when I asked him if I could give his patient a massage. Yet when I followed-up with the question, "do you mind if I apply lotion onto his back in order to offset the drying, side effects of chemotherapy and radiation, the doctor said, "Oh sure, that's fine." I simply smiled.

Cancer is just one of many "never do this" conditions that were contraindicated when I went to massage school. I get the feeling that some massage schools are afraid their graduates are going to kill or permanently maim people with massage. True, it is always possible that you could injure a client, but not if you truly think about why and what you are doing. Therapists need to think for themselves. There are no "always" and "never" scenarios in massage therapy. We need to ask ourselves one question when working with any pathology: What is the client's condition and how does a specific technique affect the client's body and their specific pathology?

Boundaries

As I have traveled throughout the United States, I have rolled my eyes more than a few times as therapists tell me that their spa tells them to "never touch" the massage table because it is the "client's domain." Or to keep one foot on the ground as you work because if you are on the table, for leverage purposes, there is a sexual connotation to the position. Wrong assumptions on both counts.

The table is a *tool* for treating clients. It is *your* tool. The client's body is the client's domain and they pay *you* and give *you* their permission to affect that domain. I mean seriously?! You can touch the client's body but not your own table? That is faulty logic. As for getting on the table in order to perform a deep tissue technique, communication is key. As long as you do not hover over the client and make them feel claustrophobic, you can be fairly confident that the treatment result is paramount and the method is up for discussion with the client.

Other therapists have been told it is "unethical" to massage above the mid thigh. From where does that line of thinking come? When I was in massage school, the owner told a story about a new client he had when he worked as a massage therapist at a chiropractor's office years earlier. The client was nearly 80 years of age and she had never received professional treatment massage. Early into the massage, he began to work on her gluteus muscles when the woman suddenly exclaimed, "Young man! Are there any muscles back there you should be working on?!"

"Well, yes ma'am," he responded. "Actually, this is the largest, most powerful muscle in your body." The woman allowed him to continue his work, but now with knowledge that would benefit her health.

The problem with a "don't massage this" mentality is that it is nearly always comes from a lack of education on either the therapist's or client's part. It may even be based on a preconceived idea from someone else's bad experience. Whether working the origins of the quadriceps muscles or the adductors of the leg, all associated skeletal muscles need to be worked in order to bring a body back into homeostasis.

Avoiding an area for the sake of misplaced propriety is absurd. I am not saying a therapist should force their techniques on an unwilling client. I am saying that education and communication are paramount for a balanced treatment session resulting in a balanced client. I cannot tell you how many clients, whom I have interviewed, have told me their therapist simply skipped the chest, abdomen and gluteal muscles, yet had the audacity to call it a "full body massage." Their therapist may have failed in math - just maybe.

While massage that is applied to every part of the body has health benefits, there must be an understanding on the therapist's part as to why they are massaging each area and what the intended benefit and outcomes are for the client. Without that understanding, they cannot educate their clients.

Breast Massage

While I was in massage school, I did some research about the topic of breast massage. Mind you, back in 1990, fellow students spent a great deal of time in class without clothes compared to now, more than two decades later. That said, I only have sisters and daughters along with a history of cancer in my family. I wanted to know more about how massage may or may not affect a woman's breast health.

During my final months of massage school training, I contacted the director of the massage division for the Washington State Department of Health. After I introduced myself, I posed a simple question, "Is breast massage legal?"

Her immediate response, without *any* hesitation was, "NO. It is *never* legal to massage the breast."

Her response began an hour-long conversation that ended with her granting me full permission to perform breast massage. Of course, but only within certain parameters: it had to be offered to everyone (not just certain types of women, etc.), with full, client consent obtained *before* beginning therapy, and to be sure to never massage the areola.

How did I convince the director to move from "NO" to "yes"? I simply asked "why?" I then used logic and sound reasoning in order to help her arrive at the ultimate conclusion that breast massage does greatly benefit the client.

I began, "Why can a therapist not massage the breast?

"Because it's sexual."

"What part is sexual?"

"The breast."

I continued, "Where does the breast begin? Isn't it really the nipple that is considered sexual and contains pleasure center innervation, which makes the situation sexual? The breast as a whole is really for feeding a baby and the sustaining of life, which wouldn't be considered sexual, right?"

"Well, yes."

"Director, do you know of what the breast is comprised?"

"It's a breast. Some make milk for babies."

"Actually, the breast consists of ligaments, fat, arteries, blood and lymph vessels, and a mammary gland for potential milk production. Ma'am, do you realize that the pressure of the bra, which you are wearing right now, can literally stop the flow of lymph in your breasts? This causes the toxins to be restricted to the tissue, unable to escape. Do you realize what long term exposure to toxins in tissue can do to the breast?"

"That can't be good."

"No ma'am. It is within my scope of practice per Washington State law to use lymphatic drainage techniques, to allow for the removal of toxins from stagnant tissues. My question is, if I have it within my ability, it is in my scope of practice and I can potentially reduce a woman's toxin-based cancer risk while improving her health, wouldn't that be a positive thing?"

"I hadn't thought of that," the Director said. "You're right. As long as you offer the technique to all women, make sure they have agreed to the treatment prior to receiving it and you don't massage the nipple, you are free to perform breast massage."

Women should be moving toxins from their breasts several times a week, if not daily, but paying a professional therapist for this would be a huge investment in both time and resources. Clientele paying a therapist to massage their breasts on a regular basis makes about as much sense as going to a shoe salesman to have him tie your shoes for you every day. However I do believe that therapists should train their clientele to massage their own breasts several times a week while and in the privacy of their own homes. Breast massage is absolutely necessary, and it is imperative that therapists educate their clientele on self-treatment. (Note: Please see the "Resources" section of our website for free information on breast cancer and breast massage at haasemyotherapy.com.)

Fascia's Control Over the Body

Many massage therapists who have taken classes about myofascial release (MFR) seem to have a common mantra that fascia is the culprit to most of the body's structural troubles. I disagree.

As we know, every muscle fiber is wrapped in fascia. Then groups of fibers are wrapped, then groups of groups, then the entire muscle. All muscular structures are fascia-wrapped. That said, this is where I differ from most MFR therapists. Realize that fascia may be "tight", but compared to the muscles themselves, it is like a 3-year old tugging on Hulk Hogan's shirt saying, "Hulk, I want to go this way!"

Hulk says back, "Good to know, but we are going this way."

The 3-year old may offer some resistance, but not ultimate control. The small amount of stress pulling against the muscle fiber is minimal.

While myofascial therapists say that they are working the fascial "restrictions," their work is *also* directly affecting the muscle, even though the benefit is not intended. The "inadvertent" work on the muscle is much like acupuncture. I firmly believe that much of the benefit of acupuncture is that it interrupts pain and spasm cycles in the affected tissues. It is called "dry needling" if a doctor does it. Same result.

There is clinical evidence that fascia actually has contractile ability. Does that force act with greater force than the muscle? Not according to any information that I have been able to gather. Saying that we are treating muscle but not fascia is as incorrect as saying we are treating fascia, but not muscle. If you treat one, you treat both.

Hydrotherapy

Hydrotherapy education is another key frustration for me. Undoubtedly, your school trained you to apply ice or heat for a given number of minutes, a recipe of sorts. The problem with using minutes when it comes to hydrotherapy is that you are looking at the clock and not your client.

Back in the mid 1980's, Owens-Corning came out with their "Visions" line of brownish, clear glass cookware. Their product was actually a chef's nightmare. They advertised that you could preheat your pan, turn off the heat and the pan "kept on cookin'!" How cool is that? Not very. Imagine you are cooking some pasta and the pot begins to boil over. You cut the flame off to the pan, but the pan, "keeps on cookin'" while boiling over and making a mess. The problem was in heat retention and poor conductivity.

Conduction is the ability for a material to transmit energy. Sure, a twig can transmit electricity, but its impedance (resistance, or poor ability to transfer energy) is not good. Copper is an amazing conductor of electricity and energy. It is why top chefs prefer using copper-based cookware because of the ability to control the heat with precision. Controlling that energy is the key, which brings us back to hydrotherapy.

If I were to blindfold you and put an ice cube directly on your skin, how long would it take before you felt the cold? Typically you would feel it in less than half of a second, or nearly instantaneously. However, if I asked you to lie on your stomach, then placed ten layers of dry terrycloth towels on your back and then placed a bag of ice cubes on top of that;, it would take a lot longer, if ever for you to feel the effect. Terrycloth towels make great insulators and do not allow heat or cold to transmit very well, especially when they are dry and the thickness is more than a couple of inches. Ice placed directly on the skin directly conducts the cold. Terrycloth? Not so much.

To correctly ice someone, you need to look for *result* instead of duration. After performing a deep shearing technique on any muscle, you should follow with ice massage. If you apply the ice massage to someone who has no inflammation, it will not take long until the area is numb. You could possibly even freeze and burn the skin. Clients *with* inflammation will take longer to ice properly. Here is the important part: You need to ice an area until it stays cold to the touch for at least 60-seconds after you finish icing. If you do that, you will have arrested the inflammation process and your treatment is finished. If the area begins to get warm to the touch again, before the 60-seconds are up, ice again and repeat until it stays cold for a full minute.

I once had a man volunteer to be a model while I demonstrated my deep tissue technique for the iliotibial band. The week before, he had purchased a brand new, 21-speed, street-racing bicycle. He rode over 200-miles that first week - his legs were on fire - and I could sense the heat from the inflammation. When performing "ice massage" to arrest inflammation, I use the bathroom-sized paper cups filled with water and then frozen. While most clients would only need 1/4 to 1/3 of the ice in that size of cup to stop the inflammation, my bicyclist melted-down *two* full ice cups until the area stayed cold. The point is this: If you ice based on time, you might under-ice or over-ice. Treat for result, not the clock.

Massage Lotions, Oils & Creams

It is funny how some therapists are so adamant about what they use to massage their clients. They are as loyal to their oils as high school kids are to their school's sports teams.

One morning I woke up to find dozens of pimples on my chest, right where the hair was coming out from the skin. They looked gross and hurt. Off to the doctor I went. The doctor told me that I had "folliculitis." How did I get that? And why then?

The doctor gave me a topical medication and it cleared up within a few days.

Two weeks later, it happened again. I returned to the doctor, but this time we had a short discussion as he interviewed me and was able to figure out the true cause of the pimples.

I had received a massage the day before both folliculitis outbreaks. He asked, "Did she work on your chest area?"

"Yes, deep work with her knuckles. It hurt and was yanking on my hairs."

The doctor smiled. "Go back to her office and ask to smell her oil. I'll bet you it is rancid. When she tugged on the hairs with her knuckles, the hairs pulled partially out of the follicles, allowing the rancid oil to make its way into the pores. That caused the follicles to get inflamed and form pimples."

The next day, I dropped by the therapist's office and asked her if I could take a look at the oil she was using. Without hesitation, she led me back to her treatment room and handed me the bottle. I unscrewed the lid and took a sniff. It was rancid.

"Smell this," I said as I held it to her nose.

"Oh god. That's bad. I used that on you!" She looked horrified at the realization.

"I know," I said with a half smile. "I got these pimples on my chest because of the oil. You might want to toss it and get some 'fresh' oil."

Many therapists use nut or plant-based oils on their clients long after it has gone bad. If a therapist buys it in bulk to save money, the odds are even more likely that it will have time to turn rancid.

While many energy workers claim that their oils have "essences" of life because the oils are from a "such and such" bush, the truth is the oil is dead food. Dead food rots. Rotting food equals rancid food. Rancid food is unhealthy and lacks its "essence." *If* you choose to use dead food as a massage lubricant, I suggest storing it in a dark glass container and refrigerate it. Even better, consider my two favorites.

The first is pure jojoba (pronounced "ho-ho-buh".) You can get it in unrefined/golden, or you can get the clearer refined version. Both work great. Jojoba oil is the same molecular weight as your natural skin oil, which means it does not just float on top of your skin, but actually nourishes it. It is also, technically, a wax.

Another type of massage lubricant that I use is Elta's paraffin oil. It is paraffin, not dead food. Not "natural," you say? Of course it is. It comes from this amazing planet of ours. Two things about paraffin or wax-based products: 1) They do not allow bacteria to grow and proliferate in the bottle if there is any contamination. And, 2) have you ever seen a freshness date or expiration date on a candle? Do candles go rancid? Nope. Both oils have significant shelf life and have amazing properties, not to mention that Elta's products are used in burn units to help burn patients in their recovery process. Why? It is not dead food and it does not have the properties of a Petri dish.

Lymphatic Treatment

The idea that a therapist should only work softly with

lymph because "5-grams of pressure" will flatten the lymph vessels, and therefore stop the flow is ridiculous. Granted, lymph in the skin might need softer strokes, but what about lymph vessels 2-inches deep into the body? Are *they* affected by 5-grams of pressure? Of course not. Deep lymph vessels need deep "squeegeeing" work. Imagine a tube of toothpaste from which you want to get every bit that you can. Do you brush the tube with your fingertips or do you squish it? You squish it! Start softly on people's lymph, then go deeper and deeper, and always toward the torso.

Scope of Practice

Understanding the scope of practice for massage therapists is extremely important. Even more critical if the therapist takes a continuing education workshop that teaches a subject like "chiropractic for the massage therapist" or "suspicious mole removal with a scalpel for the massage therapist." Just because you learn it, does not mean that it is ethical or legal to do it.

It is also important to understand that using *tools* or equipment on a patient is not in a massage therapist's scope of practice, like it is for physical therapists. Have you ever taken a class about hot stone therapy? Technically, most state licensing laws allow massage therapists to use hot stones in a stationary way for the application of hydrotherapy. However if they use those same stones for the purpose of deep tissue or other bodywork, they are now venturing into the realm of the physical therapist. Are states enforcing it? No. Can they? Yes.

Just because a police officer does not catch you breaking the law, it does not mean that you should try to get away with it.

Post MVA Waiting Period

It is generally believed, by most therapists, that soft tissue treatment should not commence until a specific period of time has transpired since the injury occurred. Some educators suggest at least a six to eight week wait.

What most do not realize is that we all have a "Spider Man," of sorts, ready to shoot a web of collagen, or scar tissue, at any soft tissue injury. It happens almost immediately.

I believe soft tissue treatment should begin the day that injuries are sustained. Would I use elbows on the injury victim's neck? Of course not, but scar tissue begins forming immediately following injury.

I figured this immediate treatment philosophy out on my own back in 1990. It was as a result of riding my Yamaha motorcycle from Olympia to Seattle while fully dressed in my leathers and Italian Ghibli helmet.

That helmet was awesome! It had this amazing visor that pulled itself away from my face and then rose smoothly when you flicked this hidden switch. I loved that helmet. It looked like a seamless, perfectly shaped, black,

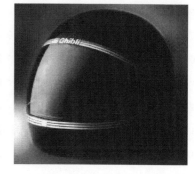

jelly bean and you could not tell what was helmet and what was visor.

While riding my motorcycle to school in the midst of a deep freeze, I banked the bike on a tight corner getting onto Interstate 5 where two on-ramp lanes merged into one. The car in front of me chose that moment to ungracefully allow the car in front of him to go first. I was following the car a bit too closely, and when he slammed on his brakes to allow the other car to pass, I had to hit my brakes, I hit a patch of black ice and my bike fell to the side taking me along with it.

All I could think about, as the bike dropped me down to the hard pavement, was that my amazing helmet was in danger of being scratched! Without hesitation, I yanked my head up, just before it skid into the ground. My suit was torn, my bike scratched, but the helmet? Pristine.

I rode my bike the rest of the way to Seattle that morning and sat through a 4-hour lecture on anatomy and physiology. Within minutes of my arrival to class, the pain in my neck began to throb. I had unilateral whiplash and it hurt, so I immediately began to work on myself. I used my hands to massage the left side of my neck using compression, cross fiber friction, and pin & stretch techniques. I treated off and on, using ice in between self-treatments during the four-hour class. I worked gently, but I was relentless. My neck hurt and all I had was time.

The next day, the pain was substantially decreased. I repeated the same protocol but with even more intensity. By the next morning, I was pain free. Just 48-hours after a severe whiplash I was out of pain.

It was not until later in my school year that I realized I had stumbled upon something. My school taught deep tissue and injury treatment, with the same mantra as most schools:

Wait. But *now* I knew better. I had experienced the benefits of immediate treatment first hand.

When I began my practice in 1991, I was able to put my theory to the test and it proved true. With every case, I observed an exponential increase in the duration of treatment versus how soon clients sought my treatment following their injuries. The bottom line is this: Start treatment immediately. Gently, tenderly, and with ice, but start it right away.

I have told my clients over the years to call me the day of an auto accident for a brief, initial treatment session. I would usually say:

"If you ever get into an auto accident, give me a call. I will squeeze you into my schedule the same day. If you call me the day of, I can perform a 10-15 minute treatment and gently start to reset range of motion, decrease inflammation and give the scar tissue direction about how to behave. If you get treatment immediately, you'll get better much faster."

Dangerous Technique vs. Cautious Treatment

As massage therapists we need to be cautious when treating in and around endangerment areas. We also need to realize that certain techniques are just outright dangerous. Let me give you a few examples.

- Many therapists are told to stay out of the triangle that is formed by the borders of the trapezius, scalenes and clavicle. That is ridiculous. *Of course* you can work inside the triangle! Just work slowly and know the structures that you are treating. For example, gently coax a scalene muscle back to health instead of giving whiplash from using excessive speed and intensity.

- While working with a client who has a compromised SI joint, be aware that putting pressure on the hip, or dropping the leg off of the table for a stretch, can cause the ligaments to sprain. These actions will destabilize the hip even further. Keep the hips square on the table as you work and use common sense about torque.

- There is a tibialis anterior technique being taught by several massage educators that is outright wrong. If the client is on their back in a supine position, pressure on the tibialis anterior needs to come into the muscle *directly*. If the client is face up (supine), and the toes of the foot are pointing at the ceiling, press into the muscle belly from a 45-degree angle, pushing the muscle back *into* the tibia bone. The incorrect method involves working the muscle with pressure along the anterior edge of the tibia bone, pushing in a posterior direction. This pulls the muscle away from the bone, giving your client shin splints. Press at a 45-degree angle instead and you will help *heal* shin splints. Deep-tracing of the posterior border of the tibia bone is equally bad as it can potentially impinge and damage the great saphenous vein. Since the bone is somewhat irregular in its formation, that allows for potential impingement and damage to the vein. Do not do it.

Migraines

I discuss migraines at length in my course, *Advanced TMJD, Head & Neck Treatment*. I will give away one secret that will be incredibly helpful for migraine sufferers.

I teach seminars throughout the country and therefore fly more often than most people and find myself inevitably working on flight attendants everywhere I go. In December of 2010, I was flying back from London when a flight attendant asked if she could get my anything. As massage therapists, we *know* when someone is in pain, even when she is trying to cover it up.

I asked, "How is your headache doing?" Her response was, "Ugh. I've got another migraine." Of course, she said it in a really nice English accent.

"Miss, does your jaw 'pop' or click when you chew?" She got a surprised look on her face.

"Yes. It's popped for years now."

"Do they have you on medications for your migraines?"

"Yes, they do."

"They don't work for you, do they?"

She gave me a look, which I often get, like I am some sort of a psychic. "No, they don't work at all."

"I'll tell you what, if you let me go to the back galley and use the gloves from your first aid kit, I'll work on your jaw, inside and out. I guarantee that ten minutes after I work on you, you will come back to my seat and tell me that your headache is gone."

Minutes later I had my gloves on and was working the muscles inside of the attendant's mouth. Her fellow attendants made a human shield of sorts, blocking us from the view of the public. I spent less than five minutes massaging the affected muscles.

Ten minutes after I returned to my seat, she stopped by. "Dear god! How did you do that? My headache is gone!"

I love hearing those words. I told her, "The reason your migraine medications do not work is because they are treating the wrong condition. You don't have migraines. You have a referred pain pattern from pain emanating from your temporomandibular joint. It's called TMJD, or TMJ Dysfunction. The pain you are feeling is an identical match to what migraines feel like. It confuses most doctors, but if the jaw is involved, the TMJ is at the root of the problem. Solve the jaw issues and your headaches will be gone. Normally, I just say, "Your jaw seems to be referring pain. I'm glad the treatment helped."

The Three-Day Headache

This next section is not so much about being a renegade, but saving a life. I will keep this short, but it is vitally important that you understand that if you ever have a client with a headache that lasts for three days, they *must* see a physician. I am not talking about a headache that lasts for 4-hours, is gone for 30-minutes, back for 6-hours, gone for 15-minutes, etc. I am talking about the headache that does not leave for at least 3-days. If a client shows up at your office presenting with this type of headache, they *may* be dealing with either an aneurism or a tumor. Have run tests run to ensure that this is not the case before you proceed with any sort of treatment.

A couple of years ago, I was riding in a cab and my attention was drawn to the back of the head of the cab driver. His head was shaved and he had a flap-cut type scar on the back of his head where the parietal bone and occipital bone meet. I asked him, "Tumor or an aneurism?"

The cab driver looked over his shoulder in disbelief. "How did you know?"

"Did you have a 3-day headache that never went away?"

"Seriously! That's so weird. How do you know this?"

"I kind of teach about this stuff for a living."

"Tumor", he said. "And yes, I had a 3-day headache."

"Do you mind telling me your story?"

"Uh, sure... I had this headache that wouldn't go away. At the end of the third day, it was getting severe and aspirin was not working. My sister insisted that we had to go to the hospital for some tests. I was not in the mood to argue. We went and the tests were performed, but the doctor said nothing was wrong. 'Like hell, nothing is wrong!', my sister said, and she took me to a hospital across town. They found a tumor in my head that day and I was immediately rushed into surgery. My sister saved my life."

What is important to keep in mind is that unless you have *two* different doctors say that there is no aneurism or tumor as the source of a three-day headache, do not continue treatment until that has been ruled out. If your client dies because you did not insist that they rule out that diagnosis, you will have a difficult time forgiving yourself. Although a massage is unlikely to be fatal, delayed testing may be.

As a side note, if a tumor or aneurism is ruled out and the headache persists, have your client ask their physician about "pseudotumor cerebri." It is a condition that mimics a tumor/aneurism type of headache and is related to an elevated cerebral spinal fluid issue. It is usually diagnosed in middle-aged women who are overweight. It is worth having their physician take another look to rule it out as well. Feel free to "Google it" when you get a chance.

Think for Yourself

The bottom line is to think when presented with a technique. Ask yourself, or better yet, your instructor, "Why are we doing this?" If the instructor cannot answer, it may require you to dust off your anatomy books and research if you are not sure.

Be sure to research from multiple sources. What is the exception to the rules of what is being taught? What is the logic behind the treatment? How do you know if it actually is doing what you are being told it is doing?

I have studied Dr. Janet Travell's work and trigger point manuals as long ago as 1990. She is now deceased and cannot defend a statement that she made, but that does not mean that I cannot reverently disagree with her. When asked 'why does putting direct pressure on a trigger point causes it to release,' Dr. Travell responded that it was because it deprived the trigger point of oxygen. In reality, it has been scientifically proven that trigger points are already hypoxic, or lacking oxygen. Her assumption was wrong. Now that you are aware, repeating disproven philosophy is a waste of time when you should be searching for the actual reason. I know *I* am still learning. And I will be until the day I die.

Pregnancy Yoga

While yoga can be a great way to relax, relieve tension and stretch, it can also be the source of lifelong, joint integrity issues, especially if performed incorrectly during pregnancy.

If a woman comes to me and states her frustration that she "feels like a bag of bones" and her joints just do not feel stable anymore, the first question I ask is if she has ever had a child. If she says "yes," my follow-up question is, "Did you take a pregnancy yoga class?" The woman usually confirms that she did.

Why is this a common occurrence? The problem is that if the woman had never taken yoga prior to being pregnant, she does not really know the limits of her normal range of motion.

During pregnancy, a hormone known as relaxin begins coursing through the veins of the mother-to-be. It is an amazingly powerful hormone that prepares the ligaments of the body, especially those in the pelvic girdle, to have flexibility in order for the baby to move through the birth canal. Yoga, or any kind of stretching for that matter, takes advantage of the relaxin and the woman could go beyond a safe range of motion. When she over-stretches, she sets herself up for a lifetime of loose ligaments, resulting in structural issues.

Once a ligament is stretched, it really does not ever return to its original length. That can be a problem. The good news is that there is a very successful treatment called "prolotherapy", or proliferant injections. To treat a damaged, weakened or stretched ligament, the doctor will usually inject a sugar-based solution directly into the affected ligament. This causes the ligament to temporarily become inflamed. The body responds by increasing the blood and nutrient supply, stimulating tissue repair, which causes ligaments to shrink back nearly to their original length, boosting joint integrity. Treatment protocols usually range from 4 to 6 sessions.

It is important to speak to your newly pregnant clients and warn them about over stretching during their pregnancy and how it can affect their joint integrity. Prevention is easier than dealing with a painful fix.

Got an Issue? Get a Tissue
(With all due respect)

Whenever someone tells me that they just received the "best full body massage" they have ever had, I ask them, "Did the therapist massage your chest muscles?"

"No."

"Did she massage your abdomen?"

"No."

"Did she massage the inner thigh?"

"No."

"Did you fail math class back in school?"

Okay, a little tongue-in-cheek, but you get my point. We toss around the term "full body massage," but are ignoring 25% of the body. The problem usually lies in the therapist's own issues that need to be addressed.

It seems that most massage therapists do not like to massage in areas that they themselves feel uncomfortable receiving massage. If they do not like their own chest worked on, they will not likely massage their client's chests. And, if they do not like to receive abdominal massage, they are not likely to massage their client's abdomens. Therapists are cheating their clients out of therapeutic bodywork because of their own issues.

Let us say that you went to a brain surgeon who had "left side issues." You sit down in front of the surgeon's desk and he tells you that he has good news and bad news. He takes a deep breath and, with a look of concern, he begins to speak.

"I am sorry to say that we have found two tumors in your brain. One on the right side, and one on the left. The good news is, I can remove the tumor on the right side. The bad news is, I need to leave the left-side tumor in place."

"Doctor, what does that mean?"

"Well, it makes *me* feel more comfortable to only remove the tumor on the right. It makes *me* feel better if I don't work on the left side. Sure, you'll likely die, but it makes *me* feel uncomfortable to work on the left side. Surely you can see that it is more important that *my* comfort comes before your health, right?"

Sound absurd? Yes. But in fact, that logic is taking place with most massages that are given on a daily basis across the country. Therapists that put their own personal comfort ahead of the client's needs are robbing their clients of optimal health. Our clients deserve a healthy and whole therapist to help them become healthy and whole. So I will say it. If you have an issue, get counseling. If you cannot offer your clients the treatment necessary to truly balance them out because of your issues, put this book down and get out of the profession.

Working as a Part of the Medical Profession

Let me be clear about one thing. Massage therapy is *not* "alternative care" and never has been. It pre-dates physical therapy and is within the scope of practice for physical therapy. Since physical therapy modalities are not considered "alternative," neither should massage be considered "alternative."

Massage therapists get into the mindset that we are alternative and therefore are outsiders to the medical profession. The only time we are outsiders is when we believe that we are. In fact, the medical profession refers to massage therapists far more than they refer to chiropractors, acupuncturists, naturopaths, or whatever else is considered "alternative."

The biggest concern that medical doctors have is that massage therapists are far from having continuity in their professionalism. I had a physician tell me once, "I would refer to massage therapists more if I knew that my patient wouldn't have to listen to sounds of whales mating while the therapist is placing crystals on them and then finish the treatment by sticking a candle in their ear." If we are to be taken seriously by the healthcare industry, we need to behave, dress, and talk like professionals.

Understanding that no healthcare professional has all of the answers is also paramount to our client's health. Chiropractors do not cure cancer. Massage therapists do not cure cancer. Oncologists, on the other hand, do treat cancer with some success. We, as therapists, *must* refer out rather than falsely believe we have the answers to all health concerns. We need to be advocates for our clients and refer them to appropriate and trusted healthcare providers. But please, for the client's sake, know what we can and cannot do as massage therapists.

Egos

There is the off chance that an ego may be involved when it comes to referring out for care. Several years ago, a friend of mine from high school called and asked if I could treat her daughter's low back pain. She found immediate relief after the first treatment. I told her that if the pain returned in two or three days, that massage alone would cure the issue and I would want to see her again before a week had passed. However, if the pain returned in two or three hours, I would need to repeat the treatment and then have her chiropractor adjust her low back within 30-minutes of the treatment.

Three hours later, she called me because the pain was starting to return. I asked her to call and schedule her daughter with her chiropractor and then let me know when the appointment was. My schedule was more flexible and I could work around the chiropractor's availability. She agreed and said she would call me right back.

Twenty minutes had passed before she called me and she sounded distraught and almost emotionally numb. "I don't know what to do. I feel caught in the middle."

I was confused. "What do you mean? What's going on?"

She went on to tell me that the chiropractor was refusing to treat her daughter if I worked on her just prior to the treatment.

I asked, "Does the chiropractor know of me and what I do for a living?"

"Yes, she's heard of you and your massage school. She said, 'If Robert Haase treats your daughter first, I won't treat her.'"

I thought for a moment. "How long has your chiropractor been treating your daughter for this specific condition?"

"Two years."

"I fear that your chiropractor is worried that if I release the spasm and then she mobilizes the joint right afterwards, that the problem will resolve. If one treatment fixes the problem, your chiropractor will be embarrassed that she has taken your time and money for the past two years for a problem that only needed a single massage treatment and just one chiropractic manipulation."

She asked, "What do I do then?"

"I've got another chiropractor that would be happy to provide that one treatment after I release the muscles."

Sure enough, just one deep tissue, quadratus lumborum/psoas release and one chiropractic mobilization later, her daughter was out of pain. The point is that you need to be aware that some healthcare providers have an ego. I am not saying that all of us do not have some level of ego involved in what we do, because none of us want to be embarrassed or look bad to our clients and patients. When referring out, speak to the other healthcare provider first and give them a heads-up as to what you are thinking. That way the "suggestion" of how to proceed can come from them and preserve their ego and hopefully help maintain a good relationship between providers.

How to Make a Quick Million Dollars

While there are some, simply amazing therapies being performed by massage therapists in the world, there are also some downright crazy ones as well.

The problem lies in the fact that some therapists will believe anything that is taught to them either in a class or seminar. I have discussed this already, but it is worth stating again: Just because it is in print or spoken by someone in "authority," does not mean it is true.

Dr. Barrie Cassileth, a researcher and educator of alternative care, is the Chief of Integrative Medicine for Memorial Sloan-Kettering Hospital in New York, NY. Dr.

Cassileth is loved by many, but there are those who wish she would keep quiet when it comes to debunking therapies that have been shown to be nothing more than quackery, including Therapeutic Touch.

At the risk of hundreds of thousands of nurses hating me, I will stand with Dr. Cassileth and say that Therapeutic Touch (TT) is pure nonsense. In case you are not familiar with TT, you might want to research it more. The "therapy" has been taught to nurses and various therapists alike since the 1970's by Dolores Krieger, RN, co-founder Dora Kunz, and those that have continued teaching her work to this day.

The basic belief is that TT practitioners can detect, assess and manipulate energy fields on the patient by merely waving his or her hands over the body. That is the short version anyway.

The problem is that a nine-year-old girl named Emily Rosa conducted an experiment that proved the therapy was not real. Her experiment, which was found to stand up to the scrutiny of the medical community, was published in *JAMA, the Journal of the American Medical Association*. It seems that young Emily conducted an experiment where 21 Therapeutic Touch practitioners   were unable to perceive her "energy field" under conditions where they would have been able to if the TT theory was valid.

The point is this: If you believe that I am wrong and you have the ability to actually discern energy fields, then pack your bags! You can be a millionaire very soon! Great news, is it not? The James Randi Educational Foundation has over $1,000,000.00 in an Evercore Wealth Management account (worth $1,285.992.96 as of April 30, 2012) and it is all yours if you can demonstrate your ability to accurately detect an energy field. Actually, the foundation is so sure that you cannot, that you can actually setup your own parameters of what skill you want to have tested. Just go to www.randi.org and look for the "$1M Challenge."

Why am I trying to discredit something that has made so many feel so good? Because it is purely placebo. As healthcare practitioners, massage therapists and touch therapists must promote good, solid science and factual outcomes if we are ever to be taken seriously. Sure, we all work "energetically," but we should not be speaking of what we are doing as factual unless it is. Again, if you believe I am clearly wrong, go get your million dollars. It is yours for the taking.

Epilogue

It has now been 23-years since I attended my first class in massage therapy. I can honestly say that embarking on this career path was the best choice I have ever made. Seeing thousands of my own clients get well, stand straighter, get back to their lives, be able to enjoy their family time again, and yes, get out of pain, has been my motivation.

As a seminar presenter, I have honed my speaking skills and have given thought more than once about using my teaching skills for other purposes. But every time I give thought to making a change, an email usually shows up in my inbox about another life that was changed due to the techniques and protocols that I teach in my seminars. It is like the old saying, "It is not about the number of apples in a tree, but the number of trees in an apple." My hope is that you will also go out and change your world, one massage at a time.

The Lights of my Life...

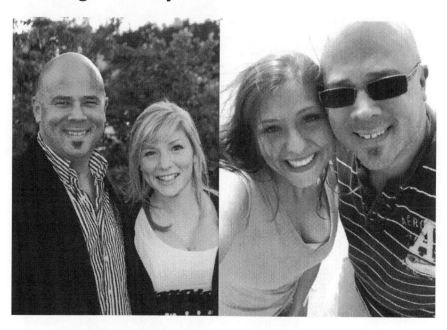

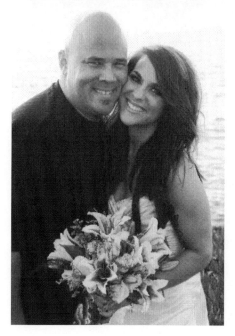

My daughters...

Top left: Sara, currently providing medical massage for a chiropractic clinic in Seattle, Washington.

Top right: My youngest, Holly, about to graduate from high school with plans for college.

Left: My oldest, Ashley, recently married and working in law enforcement.

About the Author

Raised with an all-encompassing love of art and people, Robert B. Haase was destined to be a renegade with the heart of a gentleman. As a young boy, his father gave him a camera and that gift led to a lifelong quest to share the beauty that he finds in everything. His lens captures an insightful perspective exposing others to a new way of seeing and thinking. His artistic talents were confirmed when his "Four Sirens at Breitenbush Hot Springs" won an award in the American Photo Magazine's annual, international photo contest.

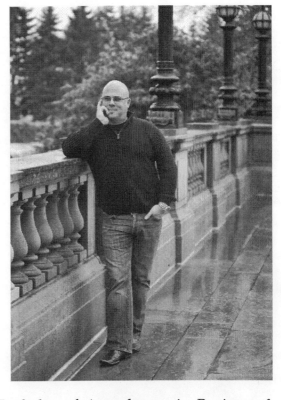

While appearing to conform to cultural "norms," Robert has earned a Bachelor of Arts degree in Business & Communications from Western Washington University along with becoming a licensed massage therapist after completing his training at Brian Utting School of Massage. Not content to be just another average massage-business owner, he developed his own curriculum and established the Bodymechanics School of Myotherapy & Massage in Olympia, WA. In the school's first year, he knew he wanted to reach out and help healthcare providers to achieve excellence in massage therapy. As a gifted speaker and entertainer he has been traveling the world teaching advanced seminars since 2001.

Robert believes in investing in the lives of individuals and his surrounding community. He has served as Marketing Director for the National Certification Board for Therapeutic Massage & Bodywork, on several boards (including The Washington Center for Performing Arts), and spoken at schools and universities. Currently he resides in Olympia, Washington near his beloved girls, Ashley, Sara, & Holly.

Made in the USA
Lexington, KY
28 December 2012